First published 2024

Perth, Australia

Enquiries to www.thewritingeditor.com.au

This is a personal memoir written by Donald Ezekiel. To the best of the writer's knowledge, memory and understanding, all names, dates and place names are as accurate as possible, but no responsibility is taken for unavoidable errors or fair presumptions.

Designed by Flametree Creative, Perth WA

Edited by Ingrid Waltham @ The Writing Editor

Published by Ingram Spark, Australia

ISBN: 978-0-6453097-5-1 (paperback)

ISBN: 978-0-6453097-6-8 (e-Book)

MY INTERESTING LIFE

A STORY OF FAMILY, FAITH AND CONTACT LENSES

DR DONALD EZEKIEL AM

CONTENTS

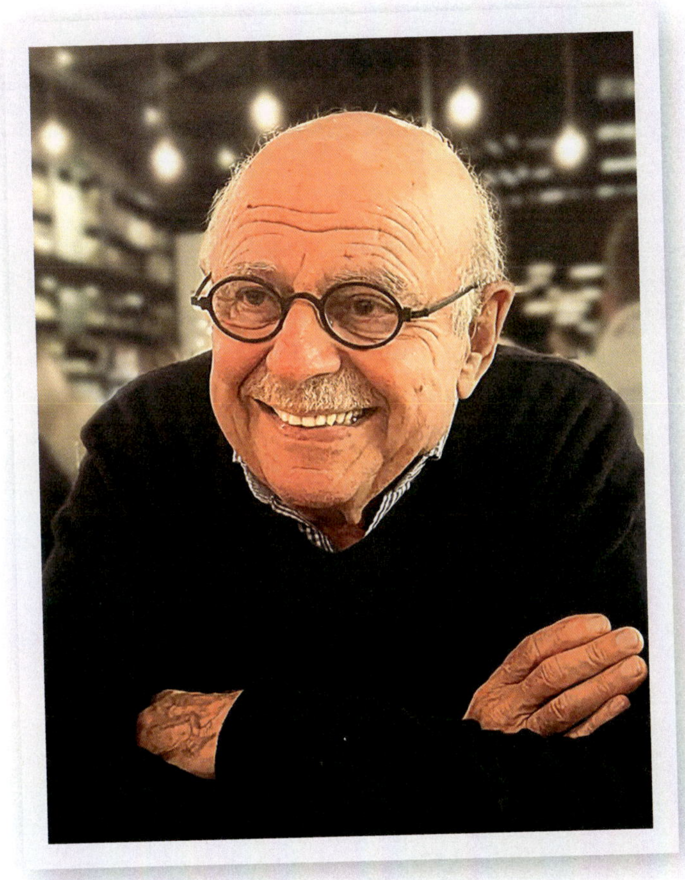

PREFACE

I was born in Singapore on 12th September 1936. This is the story of my life.

It is a memoir written for my family. It outlines what little I have managed to piece together of my parents and their family histories, together with the story of my own family and the challenges and successes that have come our way.

My parents were both refugees and neither ever really spoke about their past. I regret not having pressed them, as the experiences of their respective families would have been so interesting. Unfortunately, those stories have now largely been lost.

As well as providing an historical linkage of the family, I have also written about my career, my connections and my achievements in the contact lens industry. I was fortunate to know many of the early pioneers, including working for contact lens pioneer Joseph Dallos, who was principally responsible for encouraging me to make contact lenses. Over the years I went on to develop various lenses, some of which are used worldwide today. How these and other projects came about may be of interest to other contact lens practitioners, ophthalmologists and optometrists, and those who work in the industry.

None of this could have been possible without the support of my family, especially my understanding and supportive wife Challis, who not only put up with my crazy ideas and dreams, but has been my lovely soulmate for over 60 years. My life journey and dreams would not have been possible without her.

I truly can say I have had an 'interesting life'.

CHAPTER ONE
THE FAMILY

My Mother's Family

Due to antisemitism in their home countries, both my parents became refugees - my mother from Germany and my father from Baghdad. In 1933, aged 23, my mother left her home in Dusseldorf for Amsterdam, where she worked in a relative's department store. After her six-month visa expired, she travelled to Batavia in the Dutch West Indies (now Jakarta, Indonesia) to work for the same company. My father's family fled from Iraq to Bombay in 1920 and then on to Batavia, where he met and married my mother.

My maternal grandmother, Mutter Frieda Marks, was born on 13th May 1880 in Neersen, Gladbach. She perished in Auschwitz on 18th May 1944, after being sent there from Theresienstadt.

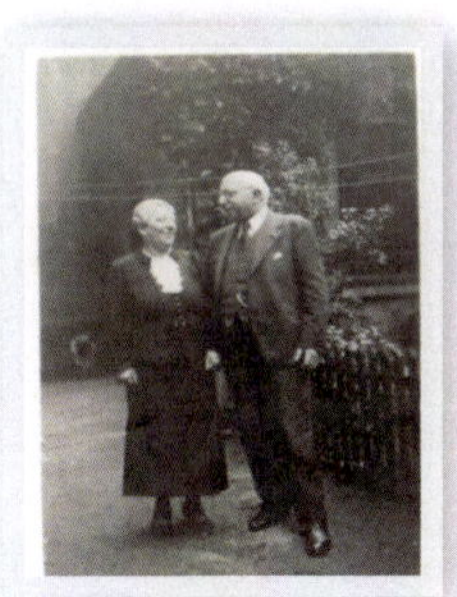

My mother's parents, Herman and Freida Hertz.

In 1963, in London, Challis and I met Tetty, a cousin of my grandmother's. Tetty told us that she was in Theresienstadt with my grandmother, and recalled witnessing my grandmother giving her rations to Tetty's young daughter.

My maternal grandfather, Herman Hertz, was born 27th August 1872 in Borghorst. He was sent to Theresienstadt on 24th December 1942, where he perished.

My nephew Guy Ezekiel obtained some chilling details about my grandfather's death.

"I contacted the Trenzishtat concentration camp. That's where Hermann Hertz died. They provided me with the attached document which shows the exact time he was burned (9:50 am). The amount of detail in the document is simply amazing. The cruelty of those people is just unbelievable." (https://spurenimvest.de/2020/10/09/marcus-anni/#comment-101)

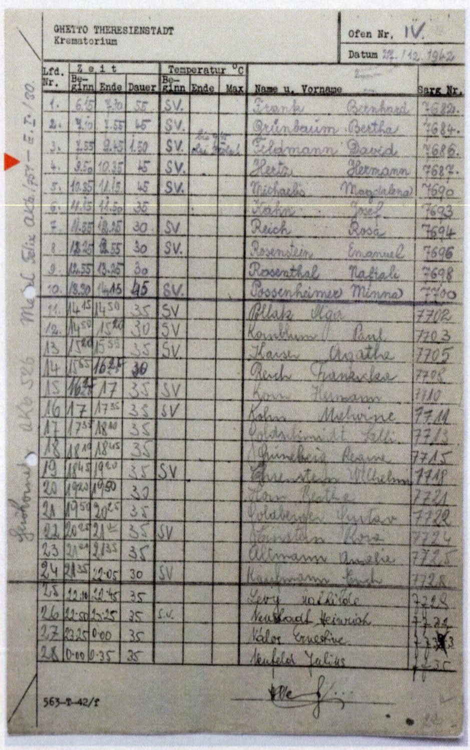
GHETTO THERESIENSTADT
Krematorium

Ofen Nr. IV.
Datum 22./12. 1942

Lfd. Nr.	Zeit Beginn	Ende	Dauer	Temperatur °C Beginn	Ende	Max	Name u. Vorname	Sarg Nr.
1.	6.15	7.30	55	SV.			Frank Bernhard	7682.
2.	7.10	7.55	45	SV.			Grünbaum Bertha	7684.
3.	7.55	9.45	1.50	SV.	[illegible]		Feldmann David	7686.
4.	9.50	10.35	45	SV.			Hertz Hermann	7687.
5.	10.35	11.15	45	SV.			Michaelis Magdalena	7690
6.	11.15	11.50	35				Kahn Josef	7693
7.	11.55	12.25	30	SV			Reich Rosa	7694
8.	12.25	12.55	30	SV.			Rosenstein Emanuel	7696
9.	12.55	13.25	30				Rosenthal Naftali	7698
10.	13.30	14.15	45	SV.			Possenheimer Minna	7700
11.	14.15	14.50	35	SV			Platz Max	7702
12.	14.50	15.20	30	SV			Kornblum Paul	7703
13	15.20	15.55	35	SV.			Kaiser Agathe	7705
14	15.55	16.25	30				Reich Franziska	7708
15	16.25	17	35	SV			Korn Hermann	7710
16	17	17.35	35	SV			Kohn Malwine	7711
17	17.35	18.10	35				Goldschmidt Selli	7713
18	18.10	18.45	35				[illegible]	7715
19	18.45	19.20	35	SV			Ehrenstein Wilhelm	7718
20	19.20	19.50	30				[illegible]	7721
21	19.50	20.25	35				Goldberger Gustav	7722
22	20.25	21.00	35	SV			[illegible]	7724
23	21.00	21.35	35				Altmann Amalie	7725
24	21.35	22.05	30	SV			Kaufmann [illegible]	7728
25	22.10	22.45	35				Levy Mathilde	7729
26	22.50	23.25	35	S.V.			Neustadt Heinrich	[illegible]
27	23.25	0.00	35				Valor Ernestine	[illegible]
28	0.00	0.35	35				Neufeld Julius	[illegible]

563-T-42/f

Crematorium document detailing the time of Hermann Hertz's extermination.

My mother was born Bertha Hertz to Herman and Freida Hertz on 4th February 1910, in Dortmund, Germany.

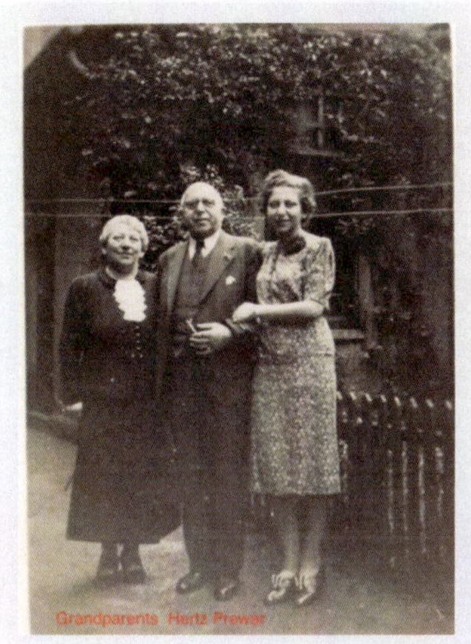

Mother with her parents Herman and Freida Hertz.

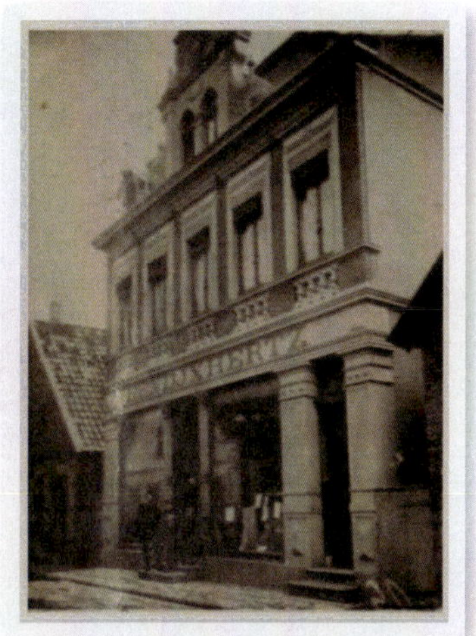

Picture of our great-grandfather's 'Hertz' house and store - the 'Hertz Borghorst' shop, where our grandparents and great-grandparents were born.

With the situation deteriorating for Jews in Germany in 1932, Bertha's parents sent her to Amsterdam in Holland (now the Netherlands) where she worked in Amsterdam's main mall in a store called Gerzon, which was owned by a relative.

My mother could only get a six-month work visa in Holland, so after six months she was sent to the Gerzon company store in Batavia. There she met and married my father, Elias Ezekiel, on 11th February 1934.

In 1938 my parents returned to Germany and tried to convince my mother's parents to leave, as it was not safe for Jews. However, her parents did not believe there would be a problem, as Germany was a civil society and her father had served with distinction for Germany in the First World War. They would not leave.

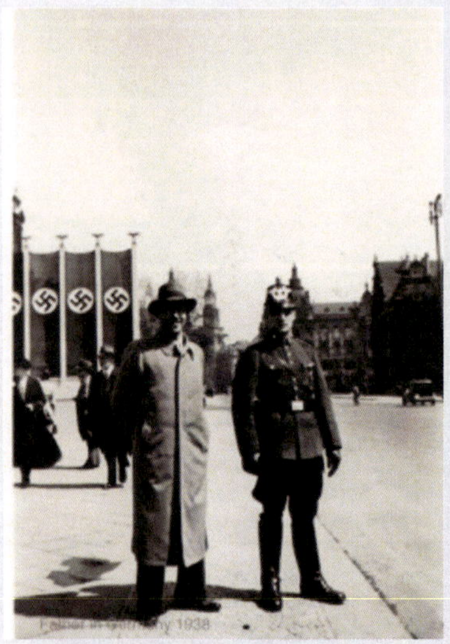

Father in Germany 1938.

My mother had a sister, Anni, who married Leo Marcus (born 16th March) 1899 in Werne.

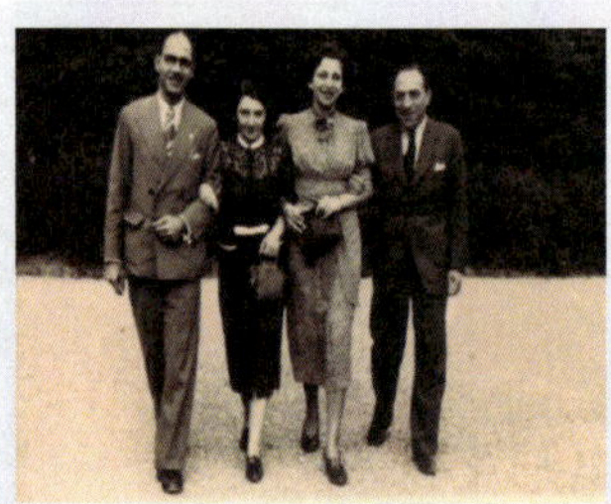

Anni and her husband Leo Marcus. They had a son Gustav, born 11th December 1934.

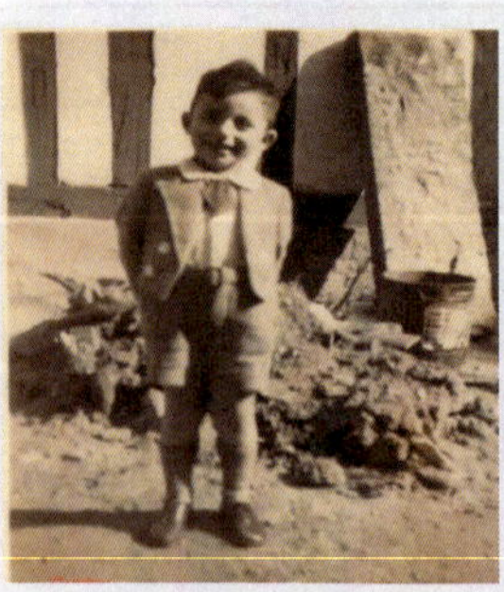

Gustav Marcus.

In 1939 Leo fled Germany for England. Anni survived the war - including three years in a concentration camp - but then spent three years after the war looking for her son Gustav in displaced persons camps.

My nephew Guy sent me the contents of a letter Annie wrote to the Jewish Information Office on Concentration Camps office in 1946. This is how it came to me - any errors are part of the original translation.

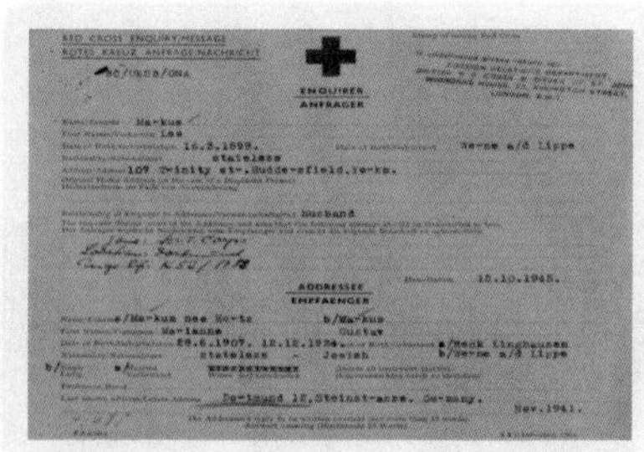
RED CROSS ENQUIRY/MESSAGE
ROTES KREUZ ANFRAGE/NACHRICHT

ENQUIRER
ANFRAGER

Ma-kus
Leo
16.5.1899.
We-ne a/d Lippe
stateless
107 Trinity st-.Hudde-sfield.Yo-ks.

Husband

15.10.1945.

ADDRESSEE
EMPFAENGER

a/Ma-kus nee He-tz
b/Ma-kus
Ma-ianne
Gustav
28.6.1907. 12.12.1934.
a/Heck Linghausen
b/We-ne a/d Lippe
stateless - Jewish

Do-tmund 12,Steinst-asse. Ge-many.
Nov.1941.

Anni Marcus Werne a.d. Lippe, 6.03.1946 at the Jewish Information Office on Concentration Camps, Munich

I am Jewish, I spent 3 years in a concentration camp, I was released by the Russians and I have been living in the city for 5 months again from which I had been evacuated.

Fortunately, my husband is in England; I already have a permission to go there. Only the formalities for departure can still take weeks.

I had only one son, Gustav Marcus, born on 11.12.1934 in Werne. He lived with me at Riga. He was deported to Auschwitz on November 2, 1943, with a mixed convoy of about 2,000 people while I was at work. I think he was gassed there. But as a mother we hold on to the slightest hope, especially since we have not attended to the assassinations and that there were survivors at Auschwitz. My husband is looking for his son worldwide, unfortunately so far unsuccessful. We did not have not yet (sic) thought about doing research in Germany.

I'm speaking to you today and asking you to have this boy searched for in Bavaria, perhaps by placing advertisements in newspapers or on the radio.

Please do not skimp on fees. I would try everything

to find it, I think you will understand. I assume that your department is responsible for Bavaria. If not, please let me know.

They are Gustav Marcus, born on 11.12.1934 in Werne, evacuated to Riga on 25.1.42 and there deported to Auschwitz on 2.11.1943. All traces of him are lost from this date. He was exceptionally tall and strong. I await your precious answer in the most promptly.

Please accept my best regards.

Anni Marcus

** stamp of receipt March 18, 1946**

Tragically, Annie never found Gustav and died of a broken heart in a mental hospital in 1948.

My Father's Family

My father, Elias Menasha (Ben David) Ezekiel, was born in Bagdad, Iraq, on 22nd December 1900. When he was two or three years old the family became refugees and left Iraq for Bombay, India.

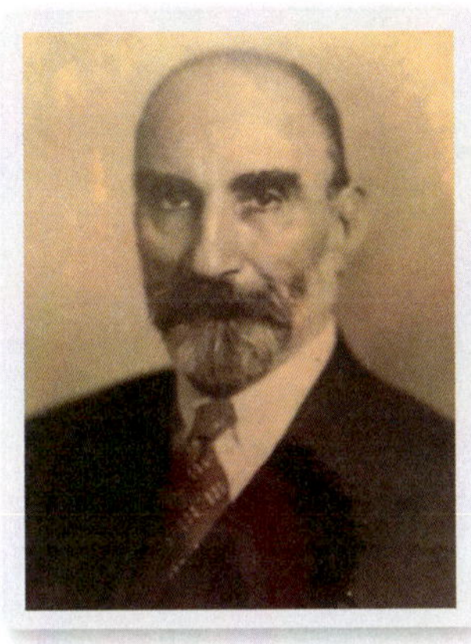

Grandfather Manasseh.

My paternal grandparents, Manasseh and Rahma Ezekiel, had five daughters - Rachel, Kesna, Kitty, Hilda and Lulu, and three sons - Charlie, Abraham (Abe) and my father Elias (Ellis). A fourth son, Ephraim, died when young. My Hebrew name is Ephraim.

As soon as they were able to, my father and his brother Abe supported the family and continued to do so for the rest of their lives. I don't think their brother Charlie ever worked.

At the age of forty, Grandfather Manasseh received authorisation by Royal Decree to settle in the Dutch East Indies. The family sailed on the ship *Rochussen* and settled in Batavia.

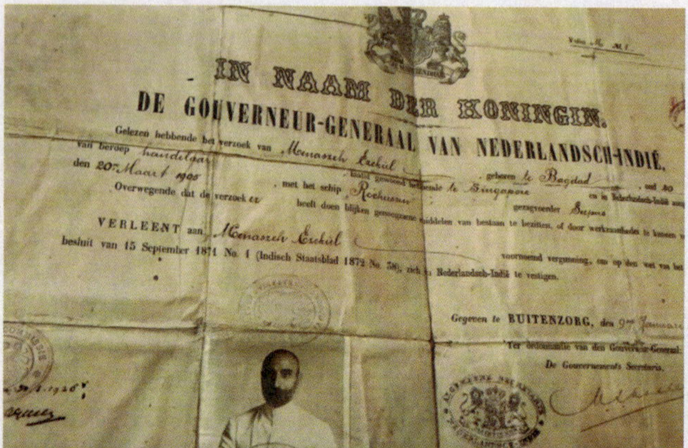

IN NAAM DER KONINGIN.

DE GOUVERNEUR-GENERAAL VAN NEDERLANDSCH-INDIË.

Gelezen hebbende het verzoek van Manasseh Ezekiel

van beroep handelaar … geboren te Bagdad

den 20 Maart 1905 … met het schip Rochussen … te Singapore

Overwegende dat de verzoeker heeft doen blijken … middelen van bestaan te bezitten, of door werkzaamheden te kunnen …

VERLEENT aan Manasseh Ezekiel … voornoemd vergunning, om op den voet van het besluit van 15 September 1871 No. 1 (Indisch Staatsblad 1872 No. 38), zich in Nederlandsch-Indië te vestigen.

Gegeven te BUITENZORG, den 9 Januari

Ter ordonnantie van den Gouverneur-Generaal.

De Gouvernements Secretaris.

A permit document allowing Grandfather Manasseh Ezekiel to move to the Dutch East Indies from Baghdad, Iraq (1905).

Official authorisation for the Ezekiel family to emigrate to the Dutch West Indies.

Abe and my father both became optometrists and established practices in Batavia and Singapore called 'M Ezekiel and Sons'. The 'M' (Manasseh) was in honour of their father.

Before he married, my father and Abe spent alternate years in the Singapore and Batavia practices. When my father married he stayed in Singapore and took over the Singapore practice.

The Jewish Historical Museum in Amsterdam held an exhibition on Jews in the Netherlands (Dutch) Indies. The Ezekiel store in Surabaya (around 1938) was included.

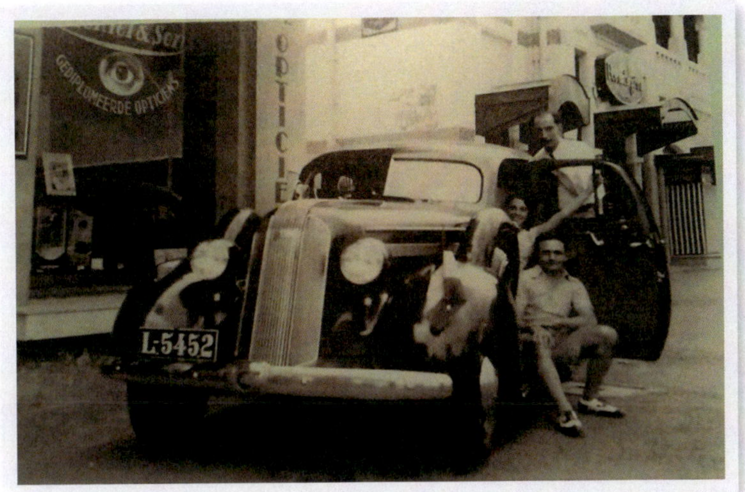

Standing is Uncle Abe. In the car is Aunty Kesner with Uncle Charlie in the foreground.

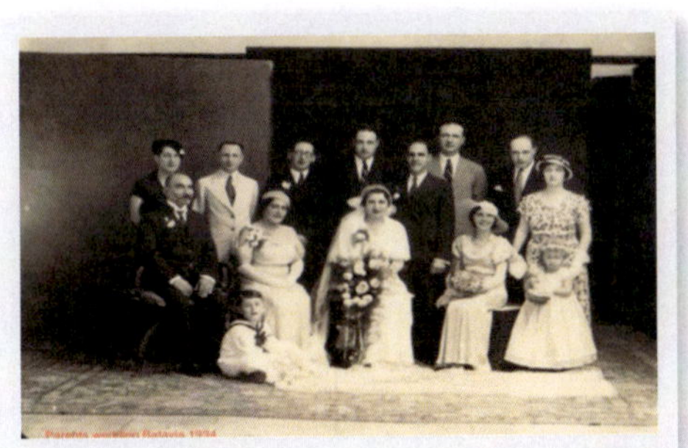

Wedding pictures of my parents Bertha Hertz and Elias Manasseh Ezekiel. Front row: Grandfather Manasseh, Aunty Rachel, mother Bertha, father Elias, Aunty Kesna.

My father and his sisters Kitty and Lulu were the only siblings who married. Kitty (Hebrew name Chatour, after her maternal mother) married a wealthy man Emanuel (Manu) Ruben on 7th October 1937. They lived in Switzerland. I don't think Manu ever worked as he inherited a substantial sum of money. They did not have any children. I don't know why but Kitty never spoke to or had any contact with my father or the family. I think she was suspicious of everyone; perhaps she felt they were after her money.

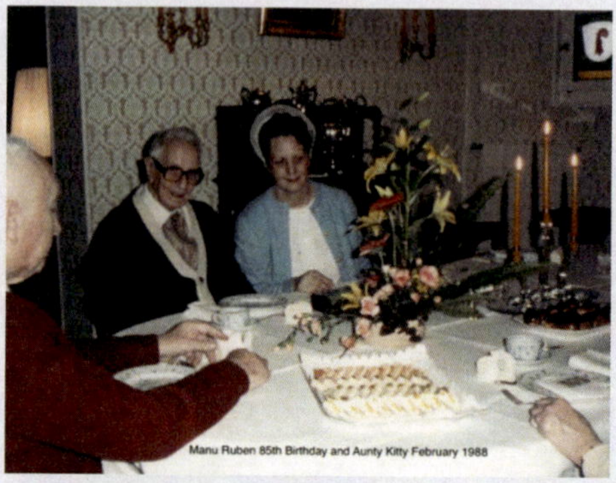

Aunty Kitty with Manu Ruben on his 85th birthday.

Challis and I visited Kitty around 1990. She was living in a five-star Swiss retirement home and we stayed there for a few days. While we were there I asked her to detail her family history for me, and she sent me a lovely letter. When Kitty died, Christies auctioned her belongings. She left Challis a lovely pearl bracelet and necklace, and my daughter Sasha a lovely bracelet.

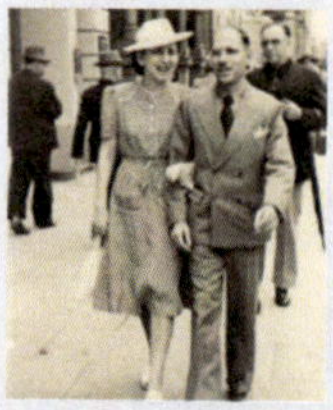

My parents in Perth during the war.

Challis's Family

Challis's parents were Mavis and James (Jim) Connell.

Mavis Philomena Kelly was born 27th July 1910, died 20th October 1984.

James (Jim) Connell was born 7th March 1904, died 4th June 1966.

They married on 27th February 1931. Jim Connell, an accountant, ran the family-owned Gosnells Hotel after leaving Wesfarmers, formerly the West Australian Farmers Cooperative.

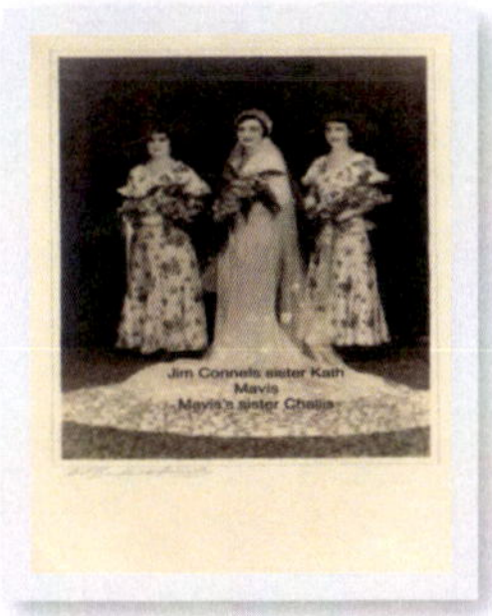

Wedding of Mavis and Jim Connell, 27th February 1931.

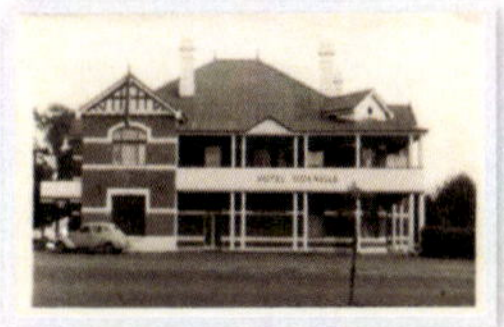

Gosnells Hotel, built in 1905 by Challis's grandfather.

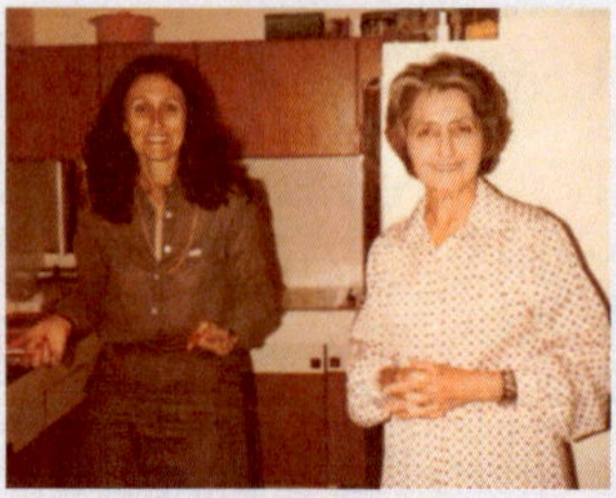

Challis with her mother Mavis Connell.

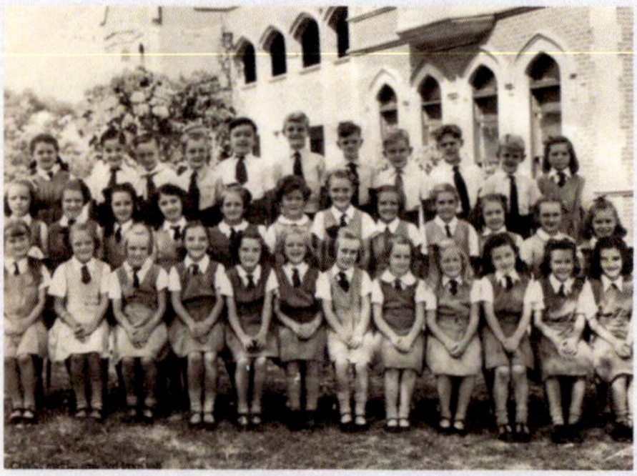

At school: Challis second row, third left.

CHAPTER TWO
EARLY YEARS

Singapore

My parents had two children. Eric was born 2nd January 1934, and I was born on 12th September 1936.

After my parents married they settled in Singapore and my father took over the Singapore optical practice. Our home was in Scots Road; my father's family home was in Katong Park. On the other side of the park was the sea. At the time, Singapore Airport was in Katong, and the road to Katong crossed the airstrip. When planes needed to use the airstrip, boom gates closed the road to car traffic.

When we visited Singapore in 2017 my cousins Frank and Mavis Benjamin took us for a drive to Katong. The house is still there as I remembered, but it is now some distance from the sea as the park has been reclaimed and built up with apartments.

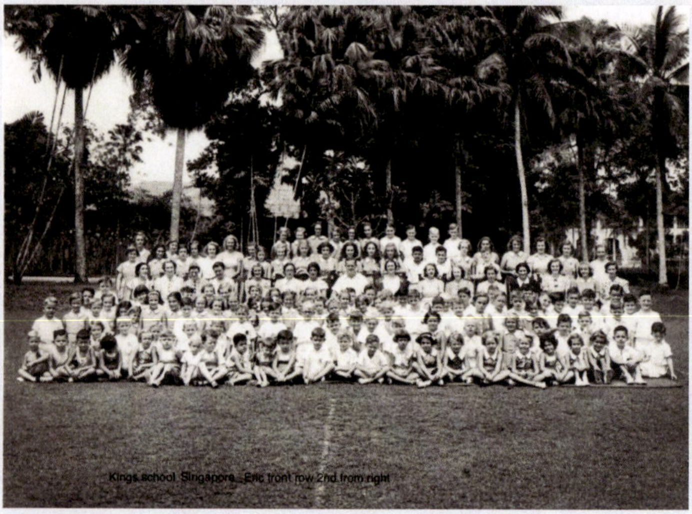

Kindergarten School
Eric and I are in the front row. I am second from the left, Eric is second from the right.

In 1942 the Japanese invaded Singapore.

Letter from Lt General Tonoyuka Jamashita to the High Commissioner of the British Army in Malaya, requesting the surrender of Singapore.

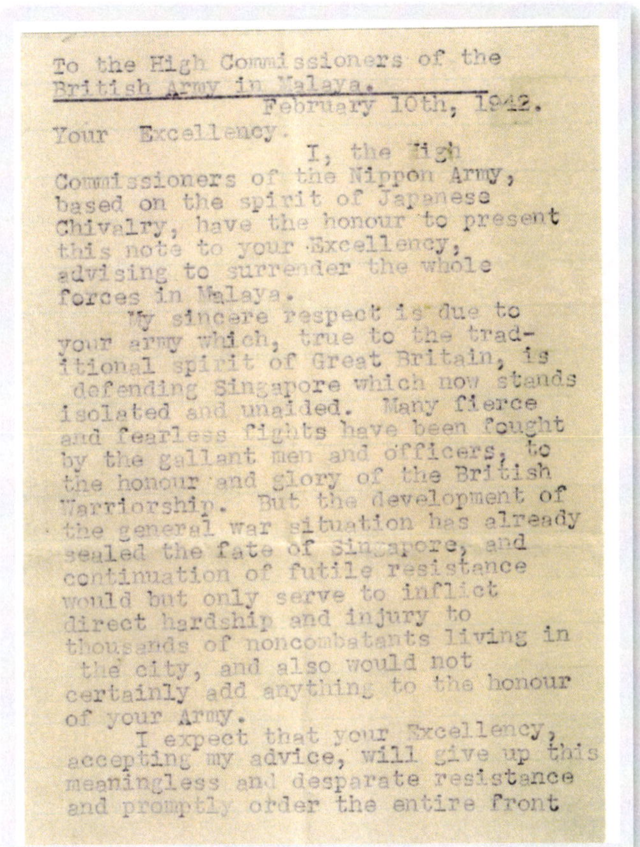

To the High Commissioners of the
British Army in Malaya.
February 10th, 1942.

Your Excellency.

I, the High Commissioners of the Nippon Army, based on the spirit of Japanese Chivalry, have the honour to present this note to your Excellency, advising to surrender the whole forces in Malaya.

My sincere respect is due to your army which, true to the traditional spirit of Great Britain, is defending Singapore which now stands isolated and unaided. Many fierce and fearless fights have been fought by the gallant men and officers, to the honour and glory of the British Warriorship. But the development of the general war situation has already sealed the fate of Singapore, and continuation of futile resistance would but only serve to inflict direct hardship and injury to thousands of noncombatants living in the city, and also would not certainly add anything to the honour of your Army.

I expect that your Excellency, accepting my advice, will give up this meaningless and desparate resistance and promptly order the entire front

Our house in Scotts Road was built on stilts. Under the house was an air-raid shelter enclosed with sandbags. Food and water were kept in large barrels, and a bare light globe hung from the ceiling.

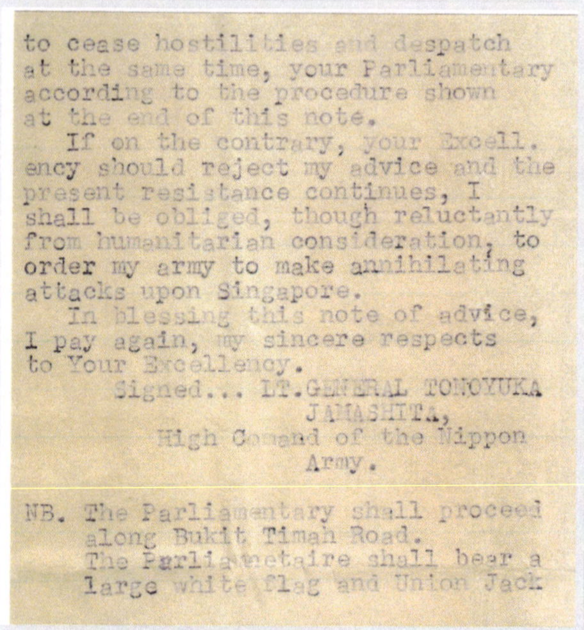

to cease hostilities and despatch
at the same time, your Parliamentary
according to the procedure shown
at the end of this note.
If on the contrary, your Excell.
ency should reject my advice and the
present resistance continues, I
shall be obliged, though reluctantly
from humanitarian consideration, to
order my army to make annihilating
attacks upon Singapore.
In blessing this note of advice,
I pay again, my sincere respects
to Your Excellency.
Signed... LT.GENERAL TONOYUKA
JAMASHITA,
High Comand of the Nippon
Army.

NB. The Parliamentary shall proceed
along Bukit Timah Road.
The Parliametaire shall bear a
large white flag and Union Jack

My mother, Eric and I managed to get on the hospital ship *Nakunda* and sailed to Fremantle, arriving on 24th February 1942. The ship had two large red crosses painted on the twin funnels, which were brightly illuminated at night. I recall sitting in a deck chair at night unaware of any danger and thinking this was lovely. Many hospital ships were torpedoed.

My father stayed in Singapore. Because his business would need to close down if he was mobilised, he was exempted from training and mobilisation on condition he joined the medical side of the passive defence services. He later managed get to Batavia and then into Australia. Beatty Saker (nee Bekhor, a Singaporean Jew who I understand is related to us through Emanual Ruben's brother) told me that her mother and her sister also managed to escape from Singapore to Perth, but her father was left behind. She told me how both her father and mine managed to escape from Singapore.

Her father had a friend who was a ship's captain on the SS *Boissevan*. He told my father to accompany him to the ship with money and he would try and get him aboard. This was successful and the ship journeyed to Melbourne. She recalled that her father told her that the trip took a long time, as the ship had to zig-zag to miss Japanese submarines and mines.

The two men both then travelled to Perth by train. Beatty remembers her family stayed at the Imperial Hotel in Wellington Street, where our family also stayed. While we were there, the phone on the wall rang. My mother answered the call. It was from my father, who had made it to Fremantle. She just dissolved in tears. It must have been hard for my mother to come to a strange country not knowing anyone.

The War Years

During the war we initially rented a house in Circe Circle, Dalkeith and later purchased a house in the same street.

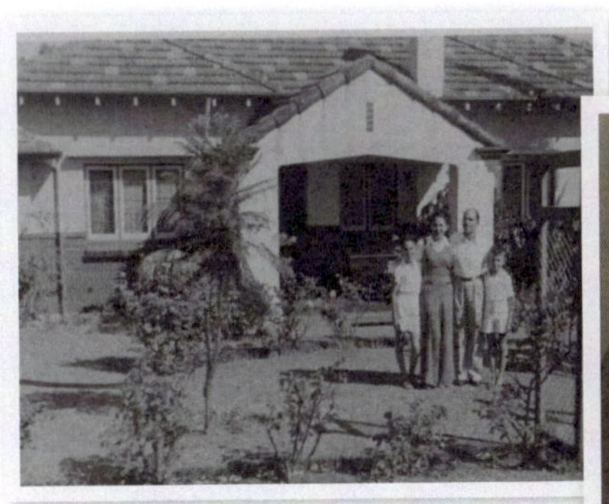

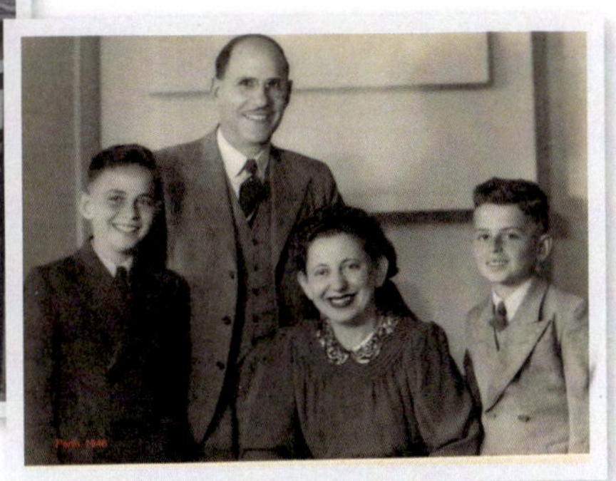

Family at home at 65 Circe Circle, Dalkeith .

Perth, 1944.

We didn't have a refrigerator, but we had an ice box where a block of ice was kept as a type of fridge. Chickens in the backyard provided us with eggs. During the war there was food rationing. I remember a truck coming to the corner of Circe Circle and Adelma Road with a load of fresh apples. We made a wooden fruit box on wheels and filled it with apples.

The shop at the corner of Adelma Road and Waratah Avenue, Warner's, was where we got our rations - including chocolate if you had the coupons. My father had a medical problem listed with the authorities, so we were allocated a ration of rice. I used to help the bread delivery man on Saturdays, delivering bread to houses on his horse and cart. My reward was a loaf of white bread, which I enjoyed eating.

We lived opposite Dalkeith State School, where Eric and I went for the early grades. When older we went to the practicing school in East Claremont. We both rode our bikes to school.

My father was an optometrist with overseas qualifications that were not recognised by the local Optometrists Registration Board. As a result he was not allowed to practice. He supported his family by welding together broken shell spectacle frames. There was a shortage of spectacle frames during the war and he would go to the city each day to collect broken frames and repair them that night. I would often sit with him as he welded the broken frames with acetone. He was an expert at repairing shell frames.

He also worked with optometrist Russell Manning in Fremantle as a technician, fitting lenses to frames and doing general optical workshop work. He tried to get registration as an optometrist but the locals did not want him in the 'club'. My father asked optometrists he knew to write letters of support to the Board, to assist in his application to practice. Some told him they would support him, but then wrote saying that he should not be recognised, and that there were plenty of optometrists in Perth and he was not needed.

The Leader of the Opposition in government at the time was Sir Ross MacDonald. He passed an Act of Parliament so that my father could practice optometry if he passed an exam. My father sat for the exam, and he passed.

My father kept all the correspondence from his efforts to get registration and compiled them into a book he called, 'Weak Eyes,

Be Wise, Ezekiel Eyes'. Eric (now with his family in Israel) has the original book. I have a copy.

My parents invited Sir Ross McDonald for dinner one night. My mother, who had never cooked a chicken before, cooked it complete - including all the intestines!

During the war people were very kind to us. The Raiters would ask us to their homes for the high holidays, and the Edelmans invited Eric and I for many Shabbat dinners and weekends when we were boarding at Scotch College after our parents had returned to Singapore. When I had my bar mitzvah, the Edelmans held a party for me at their home.

After the war my father went back to Singapore to see what he could salvage from his practice and assets. My mother followed some months later. It seems that my father's cousin Freddy Isaacs moved into his shop during the war, sold the goods and kept the money. My father took him to court to recover his losses. I think he got something back but not much. They never spoke again.

School Ships

When our parents returned to Singapore, Eric and I were sent to board at Scotch College. We would return home every Christmas for the holidays, sailing from Singapore and back on either the *Gorgon* or the *Charon*. They were called the 'school ships'. Apart from the two pursers there were no other adults on board, just school children. The food on board was great, especially after boarding school. We enjoyed the trips.

Juliet Ludbrook, who also travelled on the school ships, wrote a book about them and I was mentioned in it.

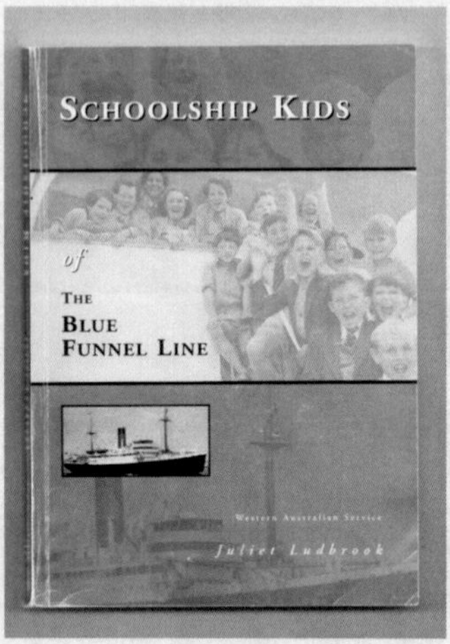

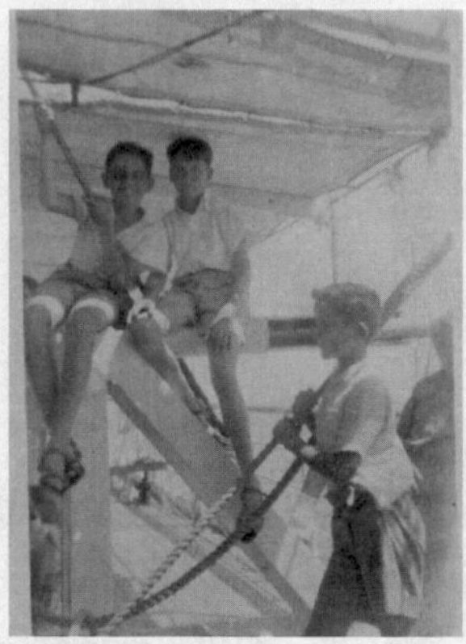

In 1949 my parents came down from Singapore for several months' holiday. Russell Manning, the Fremantle optometrist who my father worked for during the war, did a locum for him in Singapore. While they were in Perth we spent a school holiday at the Narrogin Inn in Armadale. Barry Silbert and his family were there and we became good friends. We would catch gilgies (a small freshwater crayfish) in a creek and boil them in the hotel's laundry copper. Barry assured me that once cooked they were kosher!

I travelled by bus from the Narrogin Inn to learn my bar mitzvah portion from Abe Bercov, whose father was the shamus who lived next to the shul. He was a very good teacher. Later he became a lawyer for the government but got into trouble for running a call-girl agency from his work office.

Scotch College

Eric looked after me while we boarded at Scotch College.

The first day at Scotch the teacher asked my name. I said Donald. He said, "No, your real name." A few days later I remember sitting on the lawn in front of the school, crying. I was so homesick.

Our guardians were Russell and Else Manning. They were a lovely couple and very good to us. We often spent weekends at their home.

I did not enjoy my time as a boarder. The food was awful and there were no amenities at all. My first bedroom as a boarder was in a long corridor with twenty-two beds. Morning showers were compulsory with only cold water available. The shower was constantly on and we just ran through the shower.

My parents arranged for the Sanatarium Health Food Company to send us a parcel of dried fruit each week. We enjoyed a Sunday night meal in winter of pea soup. I would take out the bacon from my plate and give it to someone at the table. We always came back for more soup! Tuesday's lunch was a roast. One of the vegetables was swede. It was awful but we had to eat it all. I always kept the envelopes from our parent's mail and would place the swede in the envelope and drop it in a rubbish bin. To help make meals edible I had a tin of mustard on the table, which I would mix with water. It wasn't special but added some taste to the meals.

We would keep Passover and buy matzos. Eric would share the matzos out for each meal, wrapped in a handkerchief. After the other boarders at the table had some, there was often very little left.

When I was aged ten, a boarder kept calling me a 'dirty Jew'. I asked our guardian Else Manning (who wasn't Jewish) what I should do and she said to hit him, but to make sure to connect the first time. I did not connect well and we were both bruised - but he never called me a dirty Jew again.

We went to shul every Saturday by bus and tram. Our father wanted us to have a good Jewish education and every Sunday afternoon we went for Hebrew lessons to a Jewish guy who taught at his home near the Hebrew school. We didn't like this when our friends were enjoying time on their own or playing sport and I am sure the teacher didn't want us there either.

Several families were very good to us. Apart from the Mannings, the Edelmans were exceptional. We often went there for Shabbat and for the high holidays. Mrs Edelman was a wonderful cook and always made us welcome. She was a real Yiddisha Mama. Her cooking was fabulous and we ate well. Their son Les became a lifelong friend.

The Benjamins, who came from Burma, lived a few doors from Scotch College and we were always welcome there. They were very good to us and Mrs Benjamin's cooking was just fabulous. Their children, Robin and Seon, were at Scotch and their daughter Rita was at MLC. Robin was in my class and a good friend.

The Perth Royal Show was always a nice experience for us. We always bought the Sanatarium Health Food breakfast show bag, as these had a selection of cereals that we enjoyed supplementing our breakfast with. They also included a collection of cards to collect showing ships. One had a picture of the *Nakunda* that we had travelled on when we fled Singapore in 1942.

On school mid-term holidays we usually went to stay at farms in the south-west. One we often stayed at was the Falconer family farm in Bridgetown. Farmer Jock milked his cows and I accompanied him on his delivery rounds where he would measure the milk from a large milk urn into the customers' containers. We had a lovely time and they were very good to us.

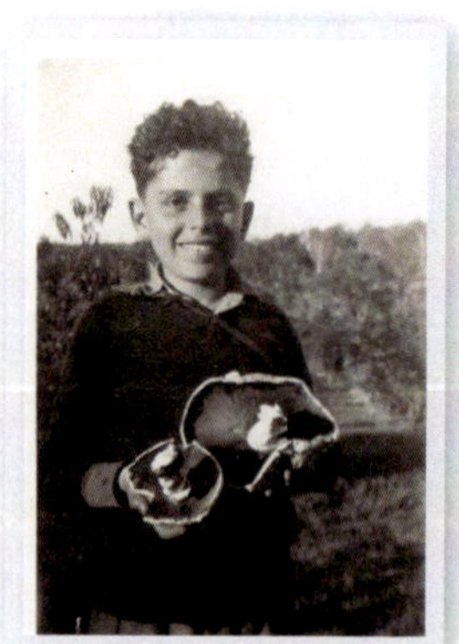

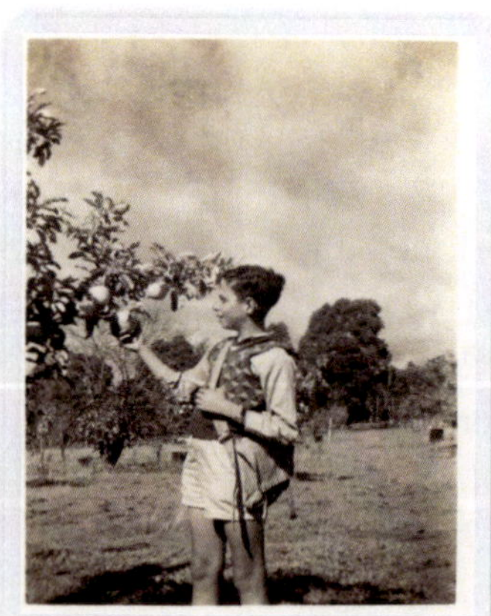

At the Falconer farm in Bridgetown.

My father's practice in Singapore was at 13 Battery Road. He built up a busy practice and did very well. My mother worked there as a receptionist and salesperson. The glass spectacle lenses were ground by an Indian gentleman called Pollani. He had Bausch and Lomb grinding machines and used coarse abrasive sand that my father collected from the beach. It worked well.

Our Christmas school holidays in Singapore were enjoyable. Our family's Singapore apartment was in Amber Mansions, off Orchard Road. (The building has since been demolished and is now the Dhoby Ghaut MRT station). The street opposite the Raffles Hotel had the best hawkers satay in Singapore. It was situated next to a large open drain, and my mother always said it wasn't clean so would bring a plate from home to put the satay on. Invariably the satay man would wipe the plate with his not-so-clean cloth before using it to put the satay on! The satay was delicious and we never got sick. We loved going to the Singapore swimming club, where we spent hours in the water and enjoyed a plate of chips with tomato sauce afterwards.

Leaving to go back to school was always sad. Luckily for me I had a very good brother who looked after me.

On the day of our arrival back in Singapore in 1951 there were racial riots. During the war, a Dutch couple had left their ten-year-old daughter Bertha Hartog with their Malay servant to care for when they fled. After the war they returned to Singapore to find Bertha had been married off to a Malay taxi driver. Her parents applied to the Singapore High Court to reclaim their daughter. The court gave the judgement directing the girl be returned to her parents, resulting in racial riots. A curfew was in place, but my father and his driver managed to get to the wharf and get us home. Our apartment was on the first floor of Amber Mansions and we could see the Gurkhas patrolling the streets in their armoured cars.

After this my mother told my father that they had run away enough times - my mother from Germany and then from Singapore, and my father from Baghdad and then from Singapore. No more running! They sold up and moved to Perth.

CHAPTER THREE
AUSTRALIA

Arrival in Australia

We moved to 43 Thomas Street, Nedlands, when my parents returned to Australia. After being boarders at Scotch College for five years we become day boys. It was a happy change. We rode our bicycles to school every day.

I did my Leaving exams, but being lazy and not studying, I only managed to pass four subjects so had to take a supplementary exam to get to university. I had lessons with a teacher called Schenberg in North Perth. He explained physics to me logically and I easily passed the supplementary exam. This gave me entrance to the University of WA and also a scholarship, which paid for my university education.

Eric did medicine. As there wasn't a medical school in Perth at the time, the first year was in Perth and the following five years in Adelaide. We missed him while he was away.

During the Christmas holiday break I had a job as a postman in the Nedlands area where we lived. I thought this was a great job as I chatted with many folk in the area and got paid to ride a bicycle. Maybe this is what I wanted to become? My father told me 'NO!' I had to study. I studied optometry as it was a four-year course and could be done in Perth.

My father started an optical practice on the first floor of a building at the corner of St Georges Terrace and King St. He did not do at all well. After about a year a shop came up on the opposite corner and he moved there. Having a display window meant more patients, but it was still not a busy practice - although much better than in the upstairs office. The shop had a flat roof and in summer the heat was unbearable. We used to take a thermos flask filled with ice to the office to have some cool water. I did the fitting of lenses to frames there. The heater we used was a hotplate, which was on all the time. This only added to the terrible heat in the building.

National Service

In the 1950s, National Service was compulsory at the age of 18. I was in the army's University Regiment at Swanbourne Barracks. Normally National Service is for six months, but being at university we did three months over the summer holidays at the Swanbourne army camp, then a monthly weekend plus a two-week camp in Northam army camp each year for three years.

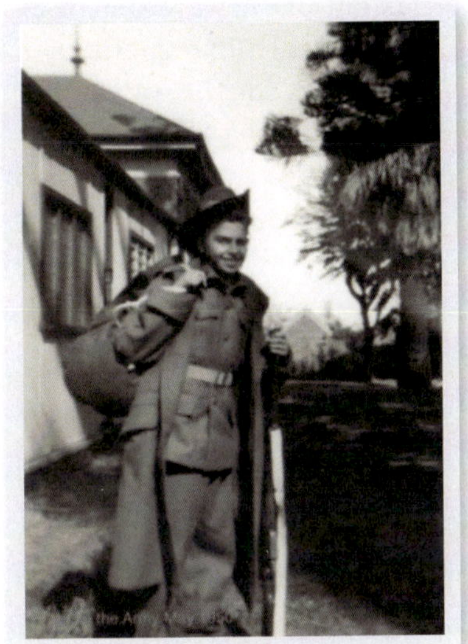

National Service.

The Jewish guys in our call-up made the most of being Jewish, and being very religious (!) we had to have Friday nights and Saturday off. This we made up by doing mess duty on Sundays.

At the end of the three months training we had a bivouac in Muchea, a bush area about fifty kilometres north of Perth. It was very hot and a bushfire had recently been through the area. It was not pleasant. I remember we all collapsed under small saltbushes and after what seemed like several hours a water truck arrived. The driver was clean and refreshed. I decided then that was the position for me, and that next time I would be driving the truck!

One thing I learned very quickly from the army was to never volunteer - no eye contact and keep a low profile. But to be an army driver I had to do a driving course in my own time. So I volunteered to do the course and became an army driver. It was well worthwhile. When we had our two-week camps in Northam I would be allotted a vehicle, made sure that the vehicle was fuelled and checked and would then locate to a hut that was not being used. I walked there with an empty file and a good book and spent the day there.

One day there was a bushfire. I was responsible for a water truck, but was busy reading in the hut. When I surfaced for lunch the camp was empty. I couldn't be found so someone else took the water truck. Back to my book. No-one missed me. Says it all!

Robin Benjamin (my old school friend) was the quarter-marshal in charge of all the camp gear located in a separate hut. Robin was a fun character and I think he got the position to keep him away from causing mischief. I often used to go to his quartermasters hut and lie on a pile of blankets to read a book. One day a senior officer came and angrily demanded to know what I was doing there, and told me not to do this again. I returned next day. We University Regiment guys spent a lot of time seeing how we could beat the system. My mother said that I reminded her of *The Good Soldier Schweick,* Jaroslav Hasek's side-splitting novel of a soldier with 'dumb insolence' under the Austro-Hungarian Empire.

Some years later when I went to renew the Australian passport I had been using for many years, I was asked if I was a naturalised Australian. I replied that I wasn't sure, but I had lived here since 1942, done National Service and just wanted to renew my Australian passport. Not good enough. I had to apply to become an Australian citizen. This I did, but declined to go to a naturalising ceremony and asked for the certificate be sent to me.

University

The optometry course was located at the physics department of the University of Western Australia. The first year subjects were with medical, physiotherapy and dental students. There were only two other students in my year at the course, Graham Fist and John Hogan.

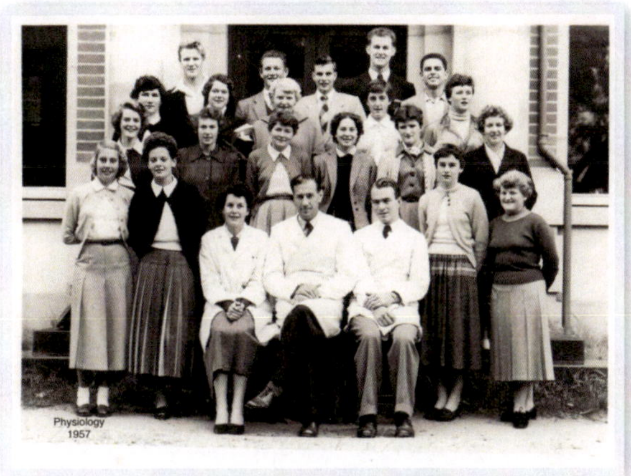

University of Western Australia. Second year physiology class.

As part of the course we had to spend time doing practical work in an optometrist practice. I worked with Russell Manning in Fremantle. He was such a nice and good man. His partner, Clive Abernethy, was in charge of the optometry course and after lectures often took me from university to their Fremantle practice. He instilled in me the importance of being professional. I well remember one Saturday morning adjusting a frame on a patient and telling him he was wise not to do this himself as he may break the frame - which I then proceeded to do. I was learning!

I graduated in 1957 with a Diploma of Optometry. Dip Opt. (WA).

Meeting Challis

For my twenty-first birthday my parents offered me the option of either a birthday party or a trip to Singapore. I chose the boat trip.

So in May 1957 I sailed for the twenty-one-day round trip on the Blue Funnel line ship *Gorgon* - the same ship I had travelled on as a school ship. On board was a gorgeous girl Challis Connell. The day after leaving Fremantle the ship called into Geraldton. I was on the deck with some other passengers, including Challis, as the boat docked. On the wharf to meet the ship was a friend I knew called Barry. I called out "Hi, Barry." A surprised Challis asked me how did I know Barry? Turns out he was her brother. Perth was a small world then, and everyone knew Barry!

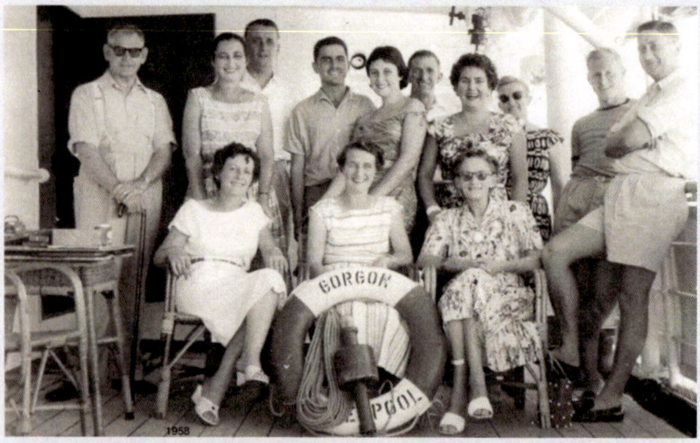

Passengers on the Gorgon 1957, Challis and I are in the centre of the back row.

Challis lived with her parents at the Gosnells Hotel, which her father Jim Connell ran. We dated when we got back to Perth but as Challis was from a strict Catholic family, any long-term future was not possible.

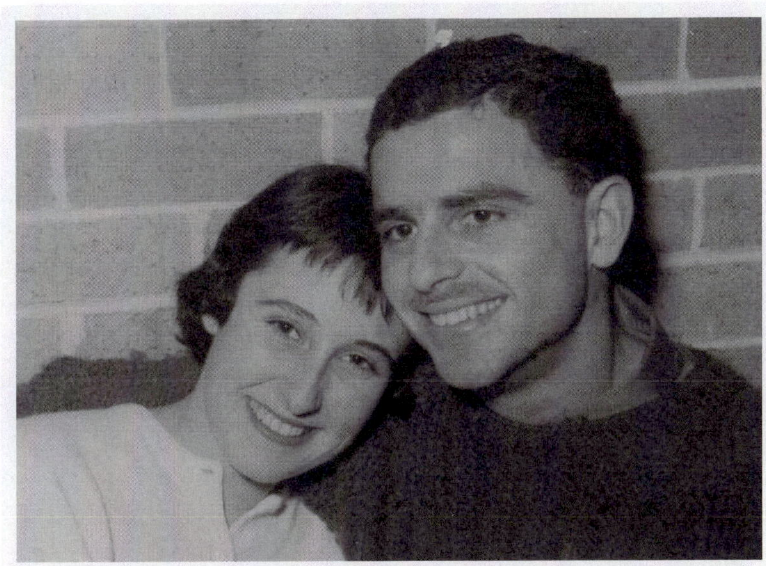

Donald and Challis.

Melbourne and Sydney

My parents were not happy with our relationship, as Challis wasn't Jewish. The flower girl at my parents wedding, Ella, was now married to a salesman, Richard Schaffer. They lived in Melbourne but Richard visited Perth twice a year, and spent a lot of time with us on his visits. He suggested that I should go to Melbourne for a year and if we were still serious after that, then my parents should accept the situation. They were not happy, but agreed.

As there was no reciprocity between the states I could not practice as an optometrist in Victoria, so I initially worked as an optical dispenser and mechanic with an upmarket shop practice in Collins Street called John Browning. Reciprocity eventually came through and I was able to practice as an optometrist. My first position was at Coles and Garrards, the largest optical group in Victoria, with branches throughout the state. Their Bourke Street practice, where I worked, had eleven optometrists on the first floor. Optometrists only did the refraction for patients. After the examination the patient was moved to a table with their record card and a dispenser took over to select a frame. One day I had a nutter of a patient and wrote on the card 'NUT++'. The patient read the card and created quite a fuss. A good lesson for me. All patient notes in future were done in code as N++!

We recorded the number of patients we saw on the day. I asked the girls in reception to pass as many patients as possible to me in the morning to get my quota up for the day - and then had a sleep on the consulting room floor after lunch. One day the boss's daughter, a Miss Walmsley, who was in charge of the testing floor, carefully opened the door of the consulting room. She saw me asleep on the floor, closed the door and never said a word. I continued my practice of an afternoon sleep.

They also had a large country practice. I often did country trips, going to a different country town in Victoria every day for the week, setting up in a room at a hotel or pharmacy and seeing patients. It was an interesting time and I learned a lot. I received a commission on all sales.

When I had moved to Melbourne Richard and Ella Schaffer arranged for me to stay in a room at the home of an Orthodox Jewish couple, Eric and Erica Weilberg. They were a lovely couple but it was a lonely time for me. I remember often having a fixed price meal at night in a restaurant in Little Collins Street. Not much, but it was cheap. I think five shillings and sixpence for a two-course meal.

I met a Jewish optometrist called Frank Kindler at Coles and Garrards and we have been good friends ever since. Frank later left Coles and Garrards and bought an old practice in Collingwood. He picked up his widowed mother every morning and took her to work with him. She always had a bacon sandwich ready for him, which we often reminded him of.

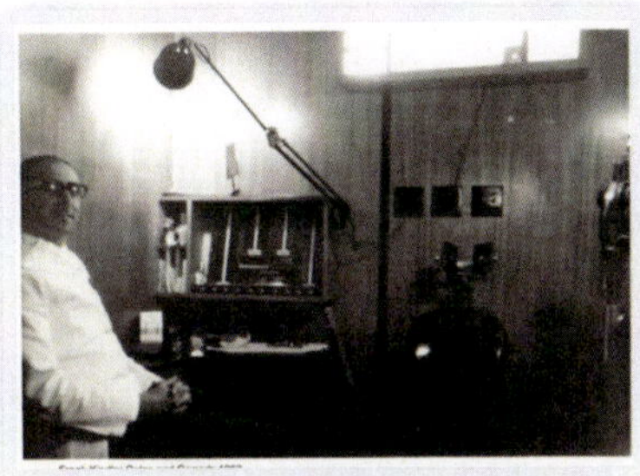

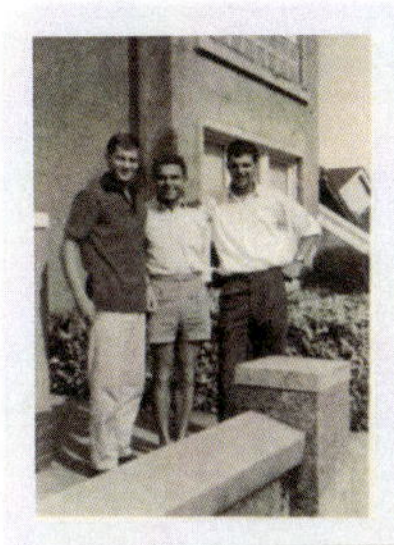

Frank Kindler at Coles and Garrards.

Elwood flatmates December 1960.

After being in Melbourne for three months, a friend from Perth, Yosse Goldberg (who was later a groomsman at our wedding) came to Melbourne and he and I moved into a flat in Elwood, together with an English fellow, Leon Godfrey. This was a very happy time.

Challis came to Melbourne to stay with some Perth girls and we continued to see each other. Before she came, I used to go to the central post office once a week to call her. As calls were cheaper after nine pm, I chatted up the fellows in charge and they would let me speak for thirty minutes for the basic cost of a three-minute phone call. I would catch a tram or hitch a ride home.

My parents bought me a Vauxhall car that allowed me to see and enjoy Melbourne. My mother came over and spent a week with me, which was lovely. Eric also visited me in Melbourne, which was great.

With Eric in Melbourne 1960.

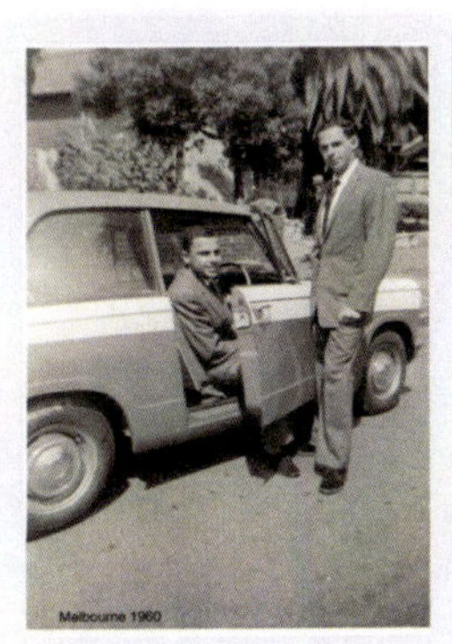

Back to Perth

I drove back to Perth, following behind a car driven by an English friend Jack Harris, known as 'Jack the Gadget Man'. Being a true novice, I was not sure if there was fuel available on the way so I carried three full drums of fuel. The road was not sealed in some parts and was just a sand track. We missed a turn-off and became bogged in a sandy area. We stayed in our cars overnight, sure that there would be traffic coming past that would help us. There was no traffic at all. Next morning I heard a tractor on a distant farm. I walked in the direction of the sound and the fellow kindly pulled us out with his tractor and directed the way back to the right road.

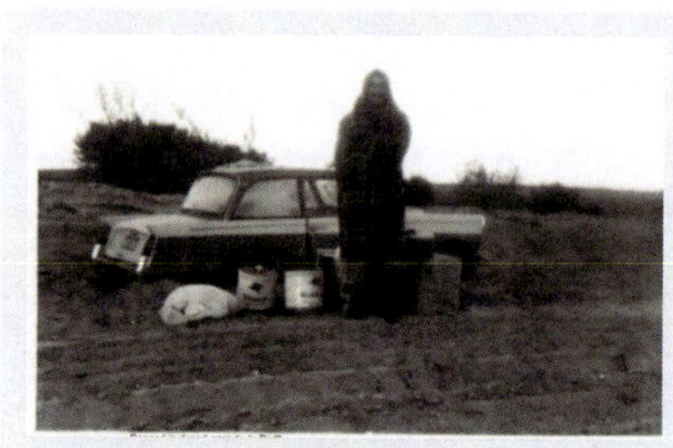

Somewhere in the Nullarbor.

Even though my father had told me I would not be welcome to work in the practice when I returned home from Melbourne, I did return to work with him. He had moved the practice from the St Georges Terrace shop to a larger shop in Barrack Street.

A lovely man called Bill Wells was our optical mechanic. As the practice was not busy I went on trips to the north-west to get some business. I had some help from the Health Department in arranging the use of hospital space to see patients.

On my first trip to the north-west I visited Kununurra, where a diversion dam for the Ord River dam project was being built. The dust was awful, it was everywhere. Apart from the workers area there was nothing; nowhere to sleep, no motel, no rental accommodation. I camped in a bed in what I thought was an unoccupied workers hut. Later that night I was wakened by the rightful occupant, so I found another unoccupied bed and slept there for the night. I was away for a month and did not do much business on that trip. Other trips were better. All flying trips were in DC3 aircrafts. It took eight hours to fly to Derby then - today it takes three!

I also visited Roebourne. As the only passenger to get off the DC3, I was taken from the airport in the back of a utility and dropped off at the hotel – because that was all that was there. Nothing moved apart for some Aboriginal people sitting under trees in the street. For two days, until the next flight out, all I did was read on a bed that was exposed on the hotel balcony. The hotel food was awful but there was no choice. There was nowhere else to eat; nothing except the one very basic pub. Some years later on another optical trip I returned to Roebourne, which by then was a bustling town. The mining boom was starting, and this time I *was* busy.

Whenever I was in Kununurra, I tried to arrange weekend trips to Cockatoo or Koolan islands. The islands are the site of iron-ore mines and were very nice. I ate in the mess with the company's office workers. With their Asian cooks, the food was tasty, especially after the terrible hotel food. One Sunday a patient took me fishing on a small boat. The fellow caught fish. I did not catch anything, even when we moved sides on the boat. He continued to catch fish and I didn't even get a bite. Nothing! Nothing has changed.

Marrying Challis

Challis converted to Judaism and we were married on 3rd January 1963 at Temple David. As the temple did not have a rabbi; we were married by Ken Arkwright. Sadly, Challis's parents did not come to the temple service, as it was not allowed at the time by the Catholic church. Challis was given away by a family friend, Doctor Emmie Kovacs. It was difficult for my parents but must have been much more difficult for Challis's parents. The reception was held at the Hotel Adelphi, a grand old hotel in St Georges Terrace that was demolished four years later.

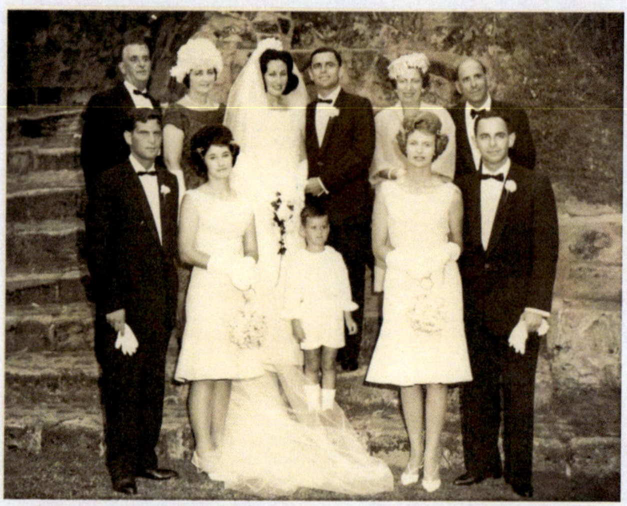

Wedding pictures. Eric was best man and Yosse Goldberg was groomsman. Bridesmaids were Bev Connell and Glennis Powell, Grant Connell was the page boy.

CHAPTER FOUR

THE UK, EUROPE AND ISRAEL

Sailing for England

Four days after our wedding, in January 1963, we sailed for England on the *Himalaya*. We had the cheapest two-berth internal cabin at the bottom of the stairs. After the first night Challis spoke to the purser, telling him the cabin was noisy and we couldn't sleep. We were upgraded to a cabin with a porthole in an area used by either first or cabin-class passengers. The English cabin steward slept in the opposite cabin. The four weeks' trip was wonderful.

I recorded details of our daily experiences in a trip book; many of the following sections are quotes are from the book.

Challis second from left, crossing the equator with King Neptune.

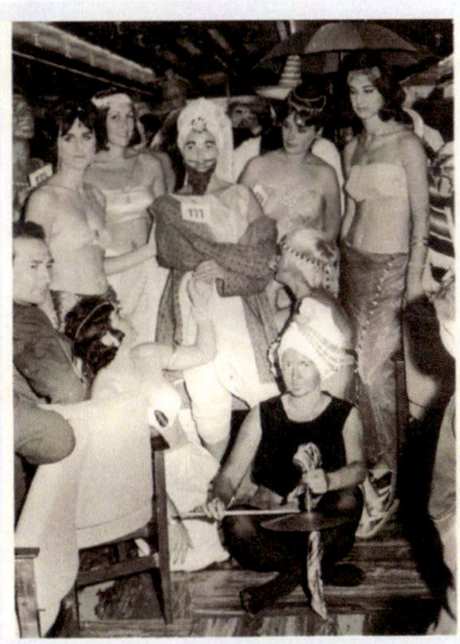

The ship stopped in Colombo, where we were told precious stones were cheap and we could make money selling them when we got to London. So we bought an aquamarine. After we paid for it, the shopkeeper gave us another stone because "we were so nice". We then realised that we had made a mistake and paid too much. We were learning!

The ship also stopped at Bombay and Marseilles. In Marseilles, the sun was out and it looked nice and warm. We debated if we should take a coat. Luckily we did as it was bitterly cold. We ate lots of delicious roasted chestnuts from a barrow on the street - but we might have had too many as we never wanted to have them again!

We arrived in London in the middle of a big freeze. The ship berthed in Portsmouth and we caught a train to London. I remember getting out from the Underground at Piccadilly Circus and it was snowing. We thought it was wonderful but were not dressed for the cold. Challis was in stockings and high heels. Before long we were both frozen. Challis had a cold that night.

We followed Frommer's book *Europe on $5 a Day* and booked into the Harley Hotel in Russell Square.

Before we left Australia we had purchased a Renault 4 tax-free to collect in Paris. As it was so cold in London that the only thing we saw was the Underground, we flew to Paris after four days to collect the car and bring it back to London. The road to Calais, where we would catch the car ferry, was iced over and the car often slid all over the road.

The ferry timetable we were given in London was the summer one, resulting in our missing the boat in Calais. The next boat departed from Dunkirk some hours later, so as we had time to spare, we browsed in shops. In one gift shop, at some distance from where we stood, a porcelain parrot with a lampshade fell and broke. The lady said we broke the lamp and told me to pay for it. I said we were not responsible for the breakage, which happened in a distant part of the showroom nowhere near us. The police were called. We still refused to pay so Challis went in the police van and I followed in the car to the police station. We were ushered into the superintendent's office to be greeted by a huge Alsatian dog chained to the desk. There was no Australian consular in Calais, so the British consul came. He told us that we were being had, but French law meant that even if he represented us and won the case, we - and our children! - may not be allowed into France again. He suggested we make an offer. I offered her 20 pounds, which was much less than the price she said the lamp was worth. She quickly accepted! I asked her for something and she gave us a porcelain doorknob. We were clearly had. Another lesson we didn't need. The British consul took us to his apartment for a strong drink. A good welcome to France, and to travelling!

When we got back to London, we needed somewhere to live. We'd heard that all Australians lived in Earls Court, so we checked the notice board at the station and rented a bedsitter. It was a large, cold room with high ceilings and a small gas heater fed with sixpenny pieces that did not make much difference. The first night we were frozen. The two single beds were of different heights but as we were so cold we put all the blankets on one bed, wore warm clothes and slept in the same bed, only to wake later in a bath of perspiration.

I went to the Northampton Polytechnic (now City University) to see if I could do a contact lens course. The head of optometry, Bob Fletcher, ran an advanced contact lens course for twelve practitioners that was booked out for a year, with a long waiting list. Bob added me to the course and I became the thirteenth student to attend the course. Bob Fletcher later became the University's Professor of Optometry.

After a month we moved to a bedsitter just behind Kilburn Station in Willesden. Our landlords, Mr and Mrs Shorn, were Jewish. They were a lovely couple and invited us for second night Seder. They lived on Regents Park in a beautiful apartment with many original paintings. It was an interesting and lovely experience for us. For the first night of Seder we were invited by Michael Wolfe, a fellow student at the advanced contact lens course. His family were Moroccan. They lived in the East End and we all crowded around a small table. It was lovely. Michael later became a professor of optometry.

The Willesden bedsit was on the first floor and had a cooking device in the room and a communal shower made in a converted broom cupboard on the landing outside. Again it ate up the sixpenny coins but the shower was great. Nice to have showers again. Our Australian friends often visited and used the shower. This was a happy time for us.

While visiting my cousin Willy Stern, we met a lady called Tetty Gartz from South Africa. She was a first cousin of my maternal grandmother, and had lived for a while with my grandparents when she was young. She had been in Theresienstadt concentration camp with my grandmother. She told me the story of how, on the first Shabbat there, my grandmother had given her bread ration to Tetty's daughter. Tetty said my grandmother was a lovely lady. I would have loved to hear more, but she was getting upset when talking about it so the subject was changed.

During this time I was studying for a contact lens exam, and Challis worked for a Harley Street specialist, a bachelor with a poodle that was looked after by his housekeeper. After a month we went to Manchester where I sat for the Fellow of the Association of Contact Specialists (FACLP) exam. We stayed with a couple we met on the ship, on beds on a veranda. It was bitterly cold! Leon Godfrey, who had flatted with me in Melbourne, had moved back to Manchester. He took us to the Whiskey a Go Go nightclub on the night before my exams. It was a fun night.

I passed the exam for the Fellow of the Association of Contact Lens Specialists (FACLP).

Bob Fletcher

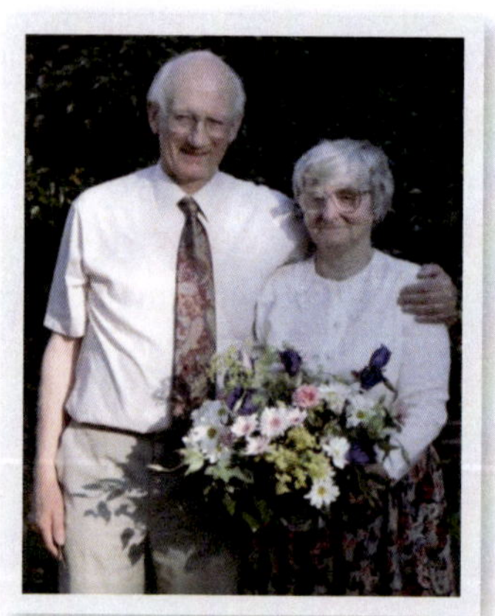

Bob and Muriel Fletcher.

The highest contact specialist exam in the UK is the Diploma Contact Lens Practice (DCLP) and was held about three months later. We decided to stay in London so that I could sit the exam. Bob Fletcher was very good to me. Before the DCLP exam he spent two-and-a-half hours giving me a private lesson. I doubt if I would have passed without his help. Bob and his wife Muriel invited us to dinner one night. They were really nice, and good people.

In 2018 I learned from a US colleague, Jan Bergmanson, that Bob had also been very good to him and suggested I could contact Bob through Bob's daughter Janet. Janet gave me their phone number and I rang and spoke with both Bob and Muriel. They were both ninety-three by then and frail. It was very nice speaking with them, and to be able to again thank Bob for giving me the opportunity with his tuition, which had enabled me to proceed on my contact lens journey. Janet copied some photos of Bob and Muriel for me. Bob looked a bit older but not changed. Muriel passed away in early 2019 and Bob passed away four weeks later.

Moorfields Eye Hospital

Through my work as an honorary optometrist at Royal Perth Hospital, I had an introduction to Moorfields Eye Hospital in north London. Frederick Ridley was the head of the hospital and greeted me warmly. He told me I should attend the contact lens clinics, which I did, witnessing pathology cases I had previously only read about in textbooks. The main lens fitter was a guy named Trode, who fitted scleral lenses in the clinic and was known for fitting a lens with a ptosis prop to hold up the upper lid. Very interesting and something I did later in my own practice. The hospital clinic was old, dark and quite primitive, with several slit lamps arranged around. Lots of protective, mainly sealed, haptic lenses were fitted, some with a groove and few ventilated. They were almost shy of the ventilated lenses. Initially focal lenses were fitted and refracted through to get the lens power.

One fitter admitted that only four hours wearing was possible with sealed lenses. The laboratory was rather ancient, but they seemed to make accurate lenses in an elaborate process. I saw many interesting cases. It was a great learning experience. Montague Reuben, who was to become the head of contact lenses at Moorfields, was a resident at the time.

Norman Bier

Norman Bier was born in Munich, Germany, in 1925 and came to England shortly before the Second World War as a refugee from the Nazi regime. He studied optometry at the Northampton Polytechnic (now City University, London) and completed examinations to become a Fellow of the British Optical Association (BOA). He subsequently gained the Honours qualification of the BOA and Fellowship of the American Academy of Optometry.

In the 1940s, only a handful of practitioners in the UK were engaged in contact lens practice but from the outset of his career, Bier dedicated himself to this specialty. A remarkable early achievement was his application in 1945 for a patent relating to the fenestration of scleral lenses.

Bier described how the fenestration of a scleral lens provided patients with all-day wearing. By accident, in the early 1940s, he realised that a scleral lens without a bubble trapped beneath it exhibited corneal oedema, while a lens that had a trapped bubble allowed longer wearing times. Building on this he developed the idea of placing a fenestration (vent) into the contact lens to enable oxygenated tears to flow into and out of the hole. It also had the advantage of reducing the pressure forces beneath the scleral lens. Bier found that a hole placed at the corneoscleral junction was adequate to provide the simple expedient of forming a bubble that moved around the limbal region upon eye movement. In combination with a minimal apical clearance and adequate limbal clearance fit, it made all-day wear of scleral lenses the rule rather than the exception.

In 1947, Bier founded Omega Contact Lens in order to fabricate his designs. In 1956, he described his contour corneal lens featuring a tri-curve back surface that was intended to provide an improved corneal fitting relationship, as compared to mono-curve microlens designs. He also invented the Bier Spherometer, the first instrument to measure the contact lens base curve, which was acquired and marketed by the American Optical Company under their trade name Radiuscope.

Bier went on to develop a preformed PMMA diagnostic set called the

Fenestrated Lens for Optic Measurement (FLOM), a system designed for US practitioners who were not allowed to use anesthetics while taking eye impressions. As gas permeable materials are heat sensitive and cannot be moulded, so have to be lathed, Norman Bier's FLOM set was ideal to establish patient fitting data to manufacture gas permeable lathed lenses. We subsequently introduced FLOM sets with Keratoconic and reverse geometry surfaces, which made the fitting of lenses for these cases much easier while taking eye impressions. I purchased a FLOM set from Omega while in London.

Bier shared his vast knowledge by publishing his first textbook, *Contact Lens Routine & Practice*, followed in 1977 with *Contact Lens Correction*, which he co-authored with Gerald E. Lowther, OD, PhD.

Norman Bier was the top contact lens practitioner in London at the time. I remember attending a lecture he gave. During the lecture Montague Reuben and a group of Moorfield doctors came in. Norman asked a question of what one would do with a particular case. Reuben put up his hand and answered: "Fenestrate the lens." Bier looked at him in disgust and said: "No. Never do that." After the lecture I asked Norman if he knew who had asked the question. He said he didn't. I told him that it was Montague Reuben, who was the heir apparent for Moorfield's contact lens clinic. "So what!" Bier replied. "It was a stupid response."

Norman Bier and his wife asked us for a Sabbath dinner. They lived in Hampstead Heath in a lovely modern home. After only seeing bedsitters and old attached homes, it was very nice to be in a normal home.

Joseph Dallos

As I needed to get some working experience – and help our budget! – I went to Harley Street in the West End, turned left into New Cavendish Street (why did I turn into New Cavendish Street?) and walked into an optical shop called Hamblins. I told them of my experience fitting contact lenses and asked if they had a position. They directed me to their contact lens clinic opposite and said that a

Dr Dallos ran the clinic, and that he was the man I should see. I was also warned that he was difficult to work with. Dallos interviewed me and offered me a job. At the interview I told him of my experience with scleral and corneal lenses. He was very nice but replied, "You don't know anything. I will teach you."

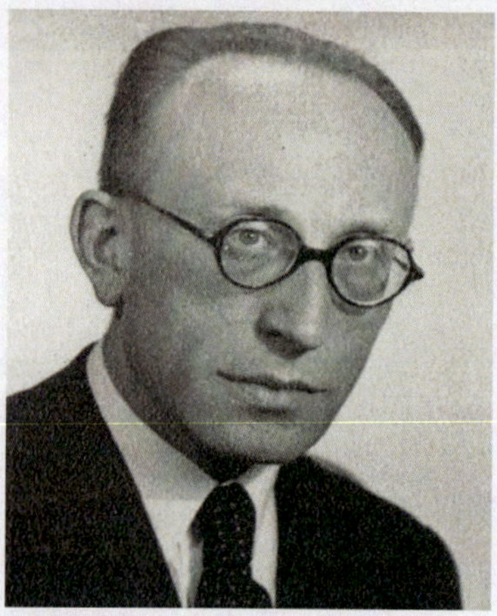

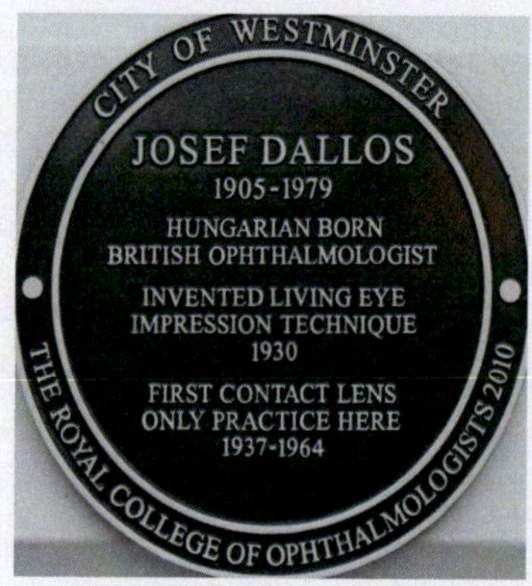

Josef Dallos.

I thought getting the job was too easy, so I phoned Bob Fletcher at the university to ask who this Dallos guy was and if it was a good place to work. Bob told me to read the first page of our university's contact lens textbook. I found out that Dallos was a pioneer in contact lenses, and the university had tried for years to get someone to learn about his fitting technique for glass scleral lenses. How lucky was I!

Although I had been told that he was a hard man to work for, we got on really well. He was like a father figure to me. I spent hours talking with him and he explained how he had made the discoveries he was famous for.

At the same time, I was offered a job at Dolland and Aitchison for twenty pounds a week. Ophthalmologist Dick Snellie, the head of Hamblins, offered me ten pounds a week. I accepted the job with

Dallos, as I thought the experience would be well worthwhile. It turned out to be a very good decision.

Dick Snellie was one of the earliest contact lens fitters in the UK to fit Zeiss lenses. He later helped Dallos settle into Hamblin's Contact Lens Centre in 31 New Cavendish Street and then to fitting Dallos lenses. This was the first practice in the UK concerned solely with fitting contact lenses.

Dallos's brother-in-law, George Nissel, established the major contact lens manufacturing machinery business at the time. He estimated that between 1937 and 1964, Dallos fitted 6,000 to 7,000 patients with scleral lenses.

At my interview Dallos asked where I lived in Australia. When I told him Perth, he asked if I knew Ida Mann, an ophthalmologist. Ida lived in the suburb of Dalkeith, just ten minutes from my family home! Dallos told me that Ida had been responsible for getting him out of Budapest and enabling him to escape the Holocaust. He asked that I pass on his best wishes when I returned to Perth. This I did, and Ida told me how she managed to get Dallos out of Hungary to London. I told her this was part of our contact lens history and asked her to document her story for me, which she was kind enough to do so. Her story is in the Appendix.

Dallos was the first person to describe how to take an impression of an eye. I asked him how he worked this out. He told me that he had a sister who was an archaeologist and that she used a dental material called Negacol to take an impression of mummies without damaging the mummy. So he thought he should try this on the human eye. His eye. From the impression taken, he would make a cast in brass, then would heat glass to mould a lens from the brass mould. All lenses Dallos fitted were made in glass.

(Later, in 2010, eye impressions were again being used. New technology developed by American optometrist Christine Sindt enabled impressions to be taken without the need for a local anesthetic. The resulting impression was scanned and the data sent to computerised lathes to accurately reproduce the front surface of the eye to the back surface of a scleral lens resulting in a perfect lens fit.)

Dallos, together with Norman Bier, were the first to describe how the 'fenestration of a scleral lens allowed for the circulation of tears from behind the lens, enabling patients to wear the scleral lens for extended periods of time'.

I asked Dallos how he had worked this out. He told me that he had a patient with areas of lens bearing at the sclera. He relieved these by grinding out these areas of lens bearing but unfortunately went through and made a hole in the lens. He polished the hole, apologised to the patient and told him he would make a new lens and to return in a week. The patient came back after several months, and when asked why he had not returned earlier, reported he did not need to come back as the lens was fine and he was wearing the lens the full day. Dallos said all he had to do then was to work out the best place to place the fenestration.

Even though he was the first to describe the taking of an impression of an eye, in all the time I worked with Dallos he never took an impression of an eye. He would always make a copy of the lens he had fitted to the patient. These lenses were then placed on three separate shelves as small, medium or large lenses. Dallos would look at the profile of a patient's eye and take a lens from the shelf that closely matched. He would then modify the lens to fit.

The practice was very basic. It had three cubicles that were curtained off with a wooden chair in each. One day he asked me to insert a lens in a child's eye. I went to the cubicle to find a three-year-old boy with an entourage of minders. I went through the motions of inserting the lens, which I was familiar with doing, but there was no way he would let me put the lens in his eye. I went to Dallos and told him. He replied, "I'll show you how to do it." He went into the cubical, picked the boy up, stood him on the chair, pushed his head against the wall and, with one hand on the boy's head and his thumb lifting the eyelid up, slipped the lens in with his other hand. He then turned to me and said, "That's how it is done," and walked out!

Over the years I have used this method many times. When my son Damon was working with me in my practice, he came into my room and told me that he was seeing a child who wouldn't let him insert a scleral lens in his eye. I said, "I'll show you how to do it!" I went to Damon's room, did a 'Dallos' lens insertion on the child, turned to Damon and said, "That's how it's done!" and walked out. I thought then that all my efforts in life had been worthwhile!

Dallos also fitted corneal lenses and never used fluorescein to assess the lens fitting of a lens on the cornea. By placing the lens slowly on the eye and looking how the lens took up onto the tear layer on the cornea he could see how the lens related to the eye and if the lens was steep, flat or a good alignment fit.

I was very fortunate to be in London at that time, as I met and knew some of the most prominent contact lens innovators involved in the development of contact lenses. These included Bob Fletcher, Montague Ruben, Norman Bier, Joseph Dallos, Frederick Ridley, George Nissel, George Gilles, Arthur Bennett, Phillip Cowdrey and David Clulow.

Life in London

We had a wonderful time in London. We went to many shows. These included Spike Milligan in *Idiot's Delight* and *The Bed Sitting Room,* which we saw twice. There was so much ad-libbing that although the shows followed the basic script, they were quite different. One quip I remember: "While I was sleeping with my partner's wife, he was in the office robbing the safe. How can one do business with a fellow like that?"

We also saw *Semi-Detached* with Sir Laurence Olivier, and the *Red Army Ensemble* at Albert Hall. We always bought the cheapest seats in the 'gods'.

Speakers Corner at Hyde Park was always entertaining. One speaker said, "The pope sent a cardinal with his blessings to Paddy Murphy, who has twenty-seven children. When told he wasn't a Catholic the cardinal was horrified. The pope had given his blessings to a sex maniac." We bought a bronze figure we called Mabel on the street on Hyde Park for nine guineas, which still has a place in our home.

I went to a European Cup Final at Wembley stadium between Benfica and Milan, standing with the crowd. It was great. It was a happy time and people were nice to us. We enjoyed going to Petticoat Lane on Sundays. Good shopping, interesting people, and great cheesecake!

On April 16 I received a letter from my father advising me that I was sacked. He had no desire to have me work with him again. I remember him writing a similar message to me when I was in Melbourne, but when I returned to Perth I again worked in the practice. Very upsetting.

I wrote to my optometrist cousin Eddie Benjamin in Singapore and he replied that I could work with him at Freddie Isaacs' practice. This would have upset my father as he had fallen out with Freddie. It was tempting to have a couple of years there. I declined, but at least I had a fallback position.

Magic

I had been introduced to magic and the local magic club by our Jewish window dresser Henry Bester. He would come to the practice and say, "Have you seen this!" and do some magic. We went to a magic studio in London called Harry Stanley, owned by magician Ken Brooks. Ken demonstrated magic and I bought close up magic tricks 'coins through the table' and a cup-and-ball routine. I went home but could not get them to work. So I went back to Ken who offered to teach me the routines for a fee, so I paid him and learned the two routines. Both are great routines, with 'coins through the table' in particular a great sleight of hand routine. When we travelled I would ask for local coins and do the routine, which often resulted in being offered a drink and asked to do it again.

I did not know at the time that Ken was a famous magician who even now has his magic online. When we returned to Perth I became a member of the Western Australian Magic Club and took part in their magic shows. I subsequently became the president of the club.

Europe and Israel

In July 1963 we left London for Europe and Israel. We had a wonderful five months touring Europe in the car and then went to Greece and Israel by ship. We stayed in some youth hostels but mainly in 'zimmer-free' pensions, or boarding houses. Our budget was five dollars a day for everything, including car costs, meals, accommodation and purchases.

We drove to Dover, caught the ferry to Bordeaux then drove to Paris. We stayed at a hotel called Hotel Marignay in Rue de Sommerrad that we found in the Frommer guide. It was run by a lovely Jewish couple. We left some luggage with them when we travelled around Europe, Greece and Israel.

We then drove to Belgium and on to Holland, where we stayed with our cousin Richard Weinberg, a relative on my mother's side. A lovely family and we enjoyed being with them and learning something of this side of our family. We then drove from Holland to Denmark and Germany. In Munich we visited Dachau concentration camp, which is in a suburb of Munich. It was very moving and on returning to our hotel we noticed some elderly gentlemen at the desk who must have known of the concentration camp.

Berlin was interesting, as it was still a divided city. One day we drove through Checkpoint Charlie to see East Germany. We declared all our cash when going through the checkpoint and drove around, always followed by a Stasis secret police car. While we were there Challis visited a toilet, for which there was a charge. Fortunately she kept the receipt, as when we returned to Checkpoint Charlie to leave East Berlin we had trouble explaining why we now had less cash than when we entered - until Challis remembered her toilet visit and produced the receipt. We were very happy to get back to West Berlin. From Germany we travelled to Austria and Venice, where we caught a ship to Greece and Israel. We left Venice on the cheapest fare I could find, on a Greek ship the *Pegasus.*

The ship was advertised as being 'air conditioned where necessary.'

There was one small air conditioner in the bar! We had travelled on the cheapest two-berth cabin on the *Himalaya*, which was nice, and we thought the same conditions would be found on this ship. This was not so; the cabin was very basic with communal bathrooms that were disgusting and the food was awful. Through Australian friends we were told of the purser they had met up with on an earlier trip on the ship. Challis went to the office and said the cabin was awful and we would like to be upgraded to a better cabin. He looked at this gorgeous girl and said, "No problem!" She told him that there were two of us travelling. Still no problem. Then I appeared ... beard and all! He was disappointed but upgraded us to first class, including meals. The ensuite shower consisted of a rusty pipe with holes running waist-high around the wall, but it was still so much better than the dirty and smelly shared amenities in economy. The food was also very much better. We spent two enjoyable weeks in Greece and then picked up the *Pegasus* again to go to Israel.

In Israel we met up with Eric and had a great two weeks with him as we travelled around the country. We were in Jerusalem for Simchas Torah. It was lovely to see people singing with Torahs in the streets.

On the ship we had met an Israeli man, Mordechai Zahera, and his wife. He is a well-known composer, and composed a song sung by Harry Belafonte. They invited us to stay with them in Tel Aviv, which we did. They were a lovely couple who were very good to us. My son Damon's Hebrew name is Mordechai.

It was sad to leave Eric. We caught the *Pegasus* back to Venice, where we retrieved the car and drove to Spain and then on to Paris to collect our luggage that we had left at the Hotel Marignay. It was now cold, and travelling in Europe was not so nice. It didn't look the same interesting place.

We drove to Genoa, shipped the car to Eric, and boarded the *Achille Lauro* for the trip home to Perth. The ship became infamous in 1985 when it was hijacked by Palestinian militants who killed a passenger, an elderly wheelchair-bound Jewish man. Some nine years later the unlucky ship caught fire and sank! Fortunately for us, it was a nice trip. We had an outside cabin with a porthole, and when we crossed the equator the King Neptune ceremony was held. As I had a beard I was King Neptune! A lot of fun.

When I reflect on how much we had seen and achieved on such a small budget and without much money in reserve, I am grateful we made it home safely.

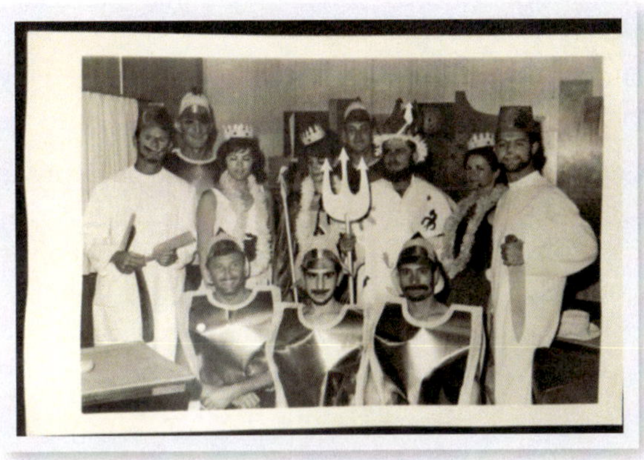

King Neptune on the way home on the Achille Laura.

CHAPTER FIVE

THE RETURN TO PERTH

The Hay Street Practice

Although my father had written to me - again - telling me that I was sacked and not welcome to work in the family practice, I did return to work there. The practice then was in Barrack Street, Perth. I started fitting contact lenses, slowly building up a contact lens specialty practice within the practice.

Some years earlier my father had opened a practice on the corner of King Street and St Georges Terrace. He later offered the practice for sale and an optical dispenser Oscar Humphries paid a deposit to purchase it. Humphries then changed his mind. I remember Humphries visiting us at home in Thomas Street, and we were sitting on the front veranda when he said he wanted to opt out of the deal. My father said fine. It was a nice thing to do.

I once went with my father to an auction of a building on the corner of London Court and Hay Street. He bought the property. Soon afterwards a Jewish guy, Mr Wilson, came in to see us at the Barrack Street practice. He had tenanted the shop in Hay Street, selling textiles. He was tearful and said he should have bought the building, and now where would he go? My father told him that he could buy the building – a decent thing of him to do.

A few years later I noticed that a building in central Hay Street was to be auctioned. I showed it to my father and stressed to him that where we were in Barrack Street, we would never be busy. We went to the auction and he bought the building. It had a common wall with the building next door, which could be a problem in the long term, so the building we bought was demolished and a new stand-alone building constructed. It was designed so that we could rent out the top floor and occupy the ground floor. We borrowed a lot of money to purchase that building. My father was not an easy person; he often changed the plans for the building for no good reason and then had them changed back, all to our cost. I did virtually all of the organising with my mother. I would go to the building site before seven am every day to check its progress and provide input of what was needed to be done. We moved to the new practice in the very best position in Perth. I spoke to a prominent ladies' hairdresser, Peter Gregory, and he rented the top floor. It was a good move and we were busy.

When we lived in Viking Road, Dalkeith, our next door neighbour was David Foukes. David managed Winterbottom Motors, a prominent car dealership, and often gave me a lift to work. I knew that they had sold their building in the city and suggested he look at a block of land my father had purchased some years earlier that ran from Adelaide Terrace to Hay Street. They purchased the property and this cleared the debt, plus gave my father cash.

Challis and I were living in a rented unit in Princess Road Nedlands, but it was too small when our second son Damon was born. My parents purchased a house at 79 Viking Road Dalkeith for us, which was so nice of them, and for us. It was a lovely home, open and bright. When Sasha was born we needed another bedroom, so we added a second floor and later a swimming pool, which we all enjoyed.

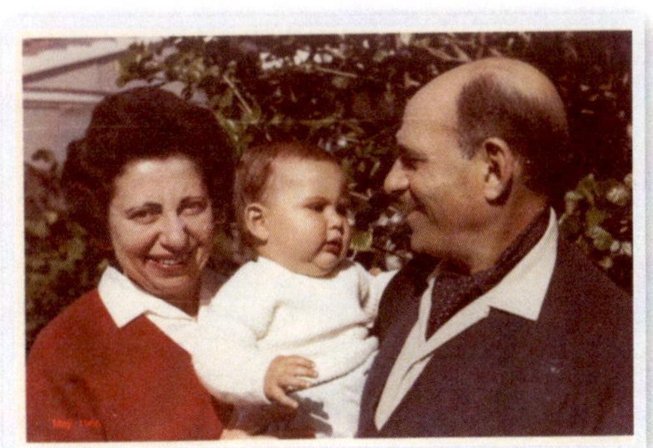

My parents with Paul.

My Mother's Illness

In 1969 my mother developed breast cancer and had a mastectomy followed by radiation treatment, which burnt her terribly. She passed away on 24th May 1971. She was a lovely, wonderful, warm, loving mother. I don't think she had a great life. Being a refugee from Germany, losing her family in the Holocaust, going to Amsterdam and then to Batavia, a strange country in the Far East, to again becoming a refugee when the Japanese invaded Singapore. Sailing on her own with two young children to a new country where she didn't know anyone, waiting in hope that her husband would follow. Returning to Singapore after the war, and then sending her children away to boarding school in Australia and missing them. Returning to Australia later in life to start again, then getting cancer and suffering badly. My father was not an easy person to live with and I don't think he was very nice to her, but she never complained.

My mother was a very warm person and got on well with everyone. One Saturday morning, the prominent English actor Warren Mitchell - famous for his lead in the TV comedy *Till Death Us Do Part* - visited the practice. I remember seeing Warren and my mother sitting on the sofa in the waiting room holding hands in earnest discussion. She was a true Yiddish mensch. When she was very ill with advanced cancer and being badly burned from radiation therapy, she would still come to the office with me to help me on Saturday mornings. My father stayed home! She always said, "Poor Dad", yet he outlived her for ten years.

I still miss her terribly.

Fallout With My Father

My father and I did not get on well. I did everything in the practice, all the ordering and most of the patient work, but I still could not do much right in his eyes. After my mother died he became quite aggressive with me. It was a very stressful time.

In 1968 I was made a minority partner in the firm and given a partnership document to sign. My father always taught me not to sign anything unless I had read it carefully. I told him that I wanted a lawyer to read it but my father made an awful scene, suggesting I didn't trust him. He took it out on my mother and she said I must trust my father, so I signed.

In 1971, about nine months after my mother died, he was getting angrier with me so I asked my lawyer and friend John Lemonis to read the partnership agreement. It read that he could buy my share back at any time for the same price I bought the share for and he could remove me from the practice whenever he wished. I went to him and told him that this did not give me security and that it needed to be changed or I would have to leave. He said no. I told him that I then did not have a choice and I would leave. He said that was okay with him. So I gave four weeks' notice. On the following Friday he lost his temper in the office in front of a busy waiting room, yelled, hit and kicked me. It was terrible. I was very upset. I phoned John Lemonis, told him what had happened and that I just could not stay. He advised me to stay to the weekend and then take my belongings and leave. So after work on Saturday morning I collected all that belonged to me that I had paid for and left my father a note saying that under the circumstances I had no choice but to not work out my notice. I said I had to leave early ... and I left.

I had not made any plans to start afresh. I had no rooms. Nothing. For a week I did nothing, as I was sure he would call me and we would get back together, as the whole purpose of the Hay Street practice was for me to carry it on. After a week with no call forthcoming, Challis found some office space on the first floor in a new building at 30 Kings Park Road in West Perth. And so I started my own practice.

Some months earlier, Challis and I had gone to Melbourne to a trade show where some German equipment, including a refractor head, chair and stand, were offered for sale at a discounted price at the end of the show. I bought it - I am not sure why, other that it was really good equipment at a really good price. Maybe fate? When I left Hay Street I took that equipment with me, along with all the contact lens records. The contact lens practice was mine; I had paid for all the necessary equipment and fitting sets needed. I paid all the bills for the contact lens business and gave the practice 50% of the takings. I had also paid for all my postgraduate training in Sydney; one thing I would always be grateful for about my father is that he stressed from an early stage of my studies that this would be the world of specialisation, and being an optometrist was just not enough. I should specialise. The training and postgraduate degrees in contact lenses that I obtained held me in good stead for the future. But although I had asked at the time if the practice would pay for my postgraduate educations and fitting sets, my father always said no.

After I left, my father immediately sent me a lawyer's letter demanding the records be returned. On the advice of John Lemonis I photocopied them and returned the originals to him. He subsequently returned the original records to me.

He then accused me of stealing, and I understand he told this to old family friends. This made me very sad as it wasn't true. I never took anything that was not contact lens related or that I had not paid for myself.

I believe that the secretary, Mrs Baker, was the problem and she turned my father against me. A few weeks after leaving the Hay Street practice I visited him at his home to 'make the peace'. We got on well. He was warm to me. It was just like old times. After about an hour with just the two of us together she came in and his attitude towards me changed totally. I never went back. The most hurtful thing was that he accused me of stealing and told our family friends. Most believed him ... at least in the early days. Those that tried to get him to reconcile with me had nothing further to do with him. Very sad as these were close friends of our family. In retrospect I now realise that he must have had early dementia or Alzheimer's. Had I realised this I am sure we would have had a relationship in his final years.

Eric, who was living in Israel, also thought that I had not behaved correctly. He did not know the true story of what had transpired. Sadly he believed the lies and conniving from Mrs Baker and did not believe me. Eric and his family even stayed with her on one of their visits and thought she was just lovely. This was very hurtful for me.

It was not until sometime later that he saw and understood what she truly was and believed my side of the sad story.

My father subsequently married (non-Jewish) Mrs Baker in the registry office. For an Orthodox Jew this was something he would never have done, let alone contemplate, in his right mind. She told her friends that she was going to get every cent and she did! What hurt me most was that we were a very close family and she divided us. I never forgave her for this. We never received any of our family's personal things when he died. It hurt. Some of our family pieces were sold from the Hay Street office. One was a Kiddush cup given to Paul for his bar mitzvah by his godparents Bev and Barry Silbert. Bev happened to see that the cup was for sale in the shop window. She bought it and gave it back to Paul.

Death of My Father

My father died on 6th August 1981. I saw him before he died, but I'm not sure he understood what I was saying to him. He left everything to his wife, his former secretary. My father's lawyer had always been Howard Solomon, but in the last year of his life I understand that his will was changed several times with another lawyer. I did not want to get hurt any more so decided not to contest the will. My brother Eric wanted to contest, as he should have been the major beneficiary. I offered to pay half Eric's legal costs for him to contest the will.

Some time before my father's death, Eric came to Perth from Israel to gather information on my father's mental health. His efforts to get any information from the doctors who cared for him was not successful, and he never continued the challenge for his rightful inheritance. Money is so evil!

Eric gave me the file of documents he gathered on my father's health condition during those last years of his life. I have since passed this onto Eric's family.

Along with the money, all the family's personal things went to his wife. It hurt us all, as she achieved what she told her friends she planned to do! I don't think that his last years living with her were happy ones for him, which is very sad as he would have loved to have had time with his grandchildren. They also missed out in not having a grandfather. Unfortunately I did not realise that he had a mental problem; if I had I might have acted differently, but I just could not take the continual knocking from him. Maybe his mental problem started much earlier, as he had sacked me on several occasions for no reason that I can think of.

Eric

Eric married Rivka in Israel on 11th August 1964. My parents went to the wedding.

Eric and Rivka had three children - Ron, Guy and Michal - and lived in a house on the beachfront in Nahariya, in the north of Israel on the border of Lebanon. Eric was a hematologist and created the blood bank in the north of Israel. Prior to the establishment of the blood bank, people only donated blood as it was needed. He told me that he often moved across the Green Line to care for Arabs in Lebanon, sitting in their tents treating and talking with them.

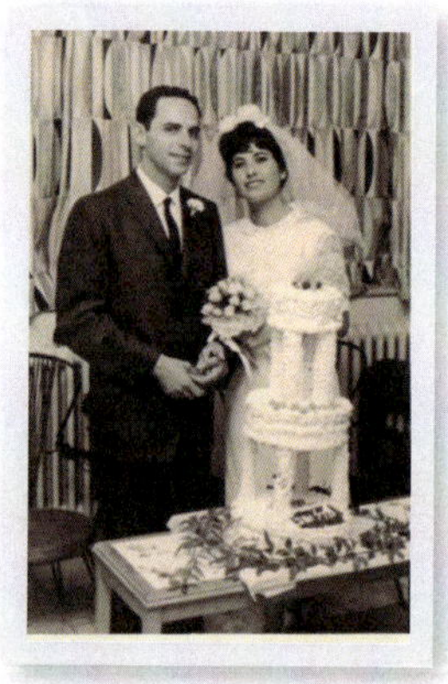

Eric and Rivka's wedding.

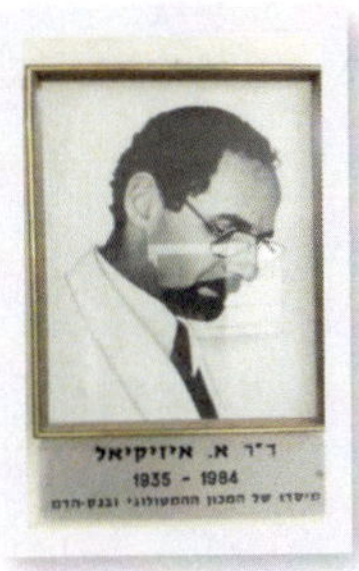

Picture of Eric prominently displayed at the hospital in Nahariya.

Sadly, Eric died of an aneurism in 1987, at the age of just forty-nine. He left a widow and three young children.

A year after his death we went to Israel for the setting of the stone. More Arabs than Jews were at the setting of the stone ceremony.

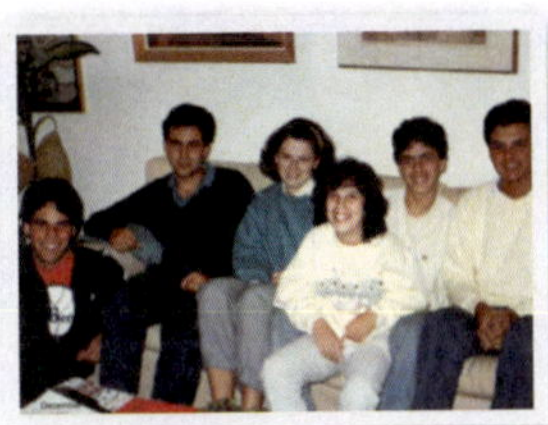

Our Israeli family.

Eric's children are all now married with children. The families are lovely. All have done well. Eric would have been very proud of them.

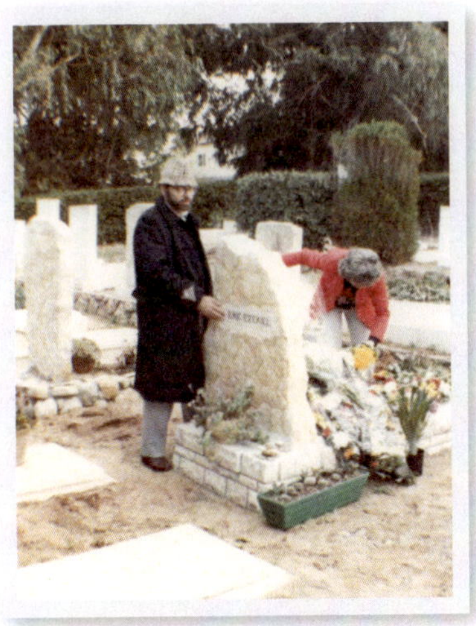

The setting of the stone a year after Eric's death.

From Israel we travelled to Zermatt in Switzerland. Paul, Damon and Sasha skied, and Challis and I walked the trails. It was lovely.

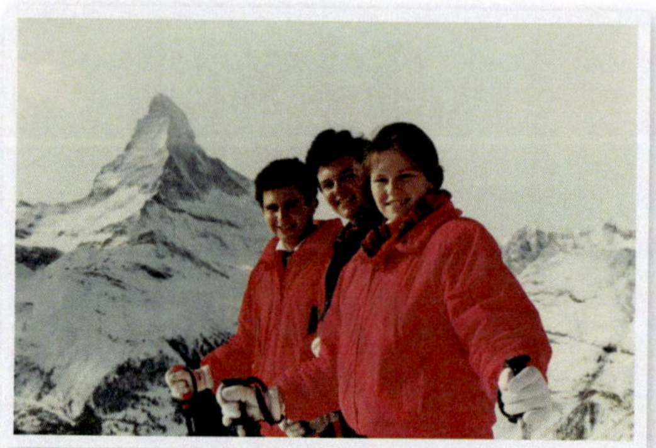

CHAPTER SIX
THE CHILDREN

Our three children.

Paul, born 1st June 1965

Damon born 16th February 1967

Sasha born 17th March 1971

Paul and Damon went to my old school, Scotch College, and Sasha went to Presbyterian Ladies College (PLC).

Paul

Paul was house captain of St Andrews at Scotch. He went on to do medicine. When he was younger, Paul would never be present if anyone was sick or had a cut, yet in the summer holidays after his first year of medicine he worked in the morgue preparing the bodies for the next year's anatomy students. Paul graduated and enjoyed medicine. Between years five and six year of the medical course, students were encouraged to do an elective term at an overseas hospital. Paul did his elective at Beth Israel hospital in Boston. He stayed with our optometrist friends Donald and Joan Korb and also with a patient of mine, Mark Barnaba, who was doing a Master of Business Administration (MBA) at Harvard. Paul phoned one day saying the MBA course sounded very interesting and that he might give up medicine and do an MBA. We told Paul to complete the medical degree and then reconsider leaving medicine and doing an MBA, which he did.

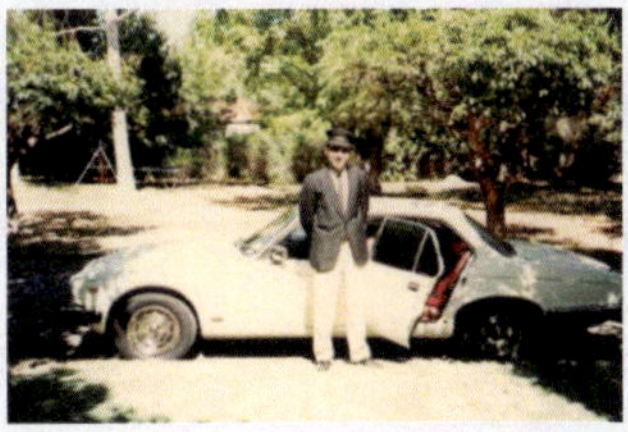

Paul as chauffeur driver during the America's Cup.

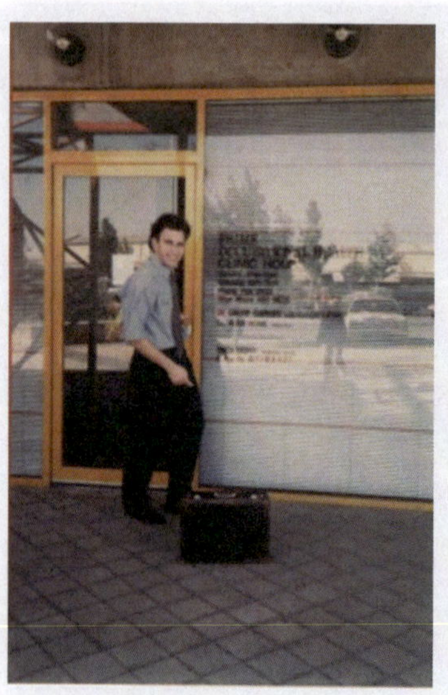

Paul working as a GP.

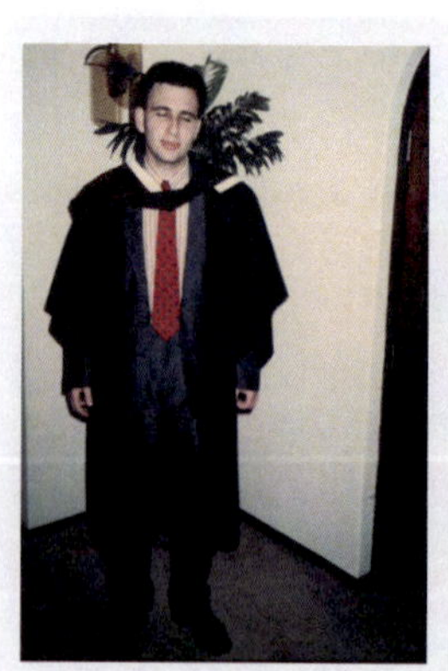

Paul graduated in medicine.

After practicing medicine for five years, where he was in senior neurosurgeon Bryan (Bars) Stokes' neurosurgery stream, he left for Cornell University in Ithaca, New York, to do an MBA.

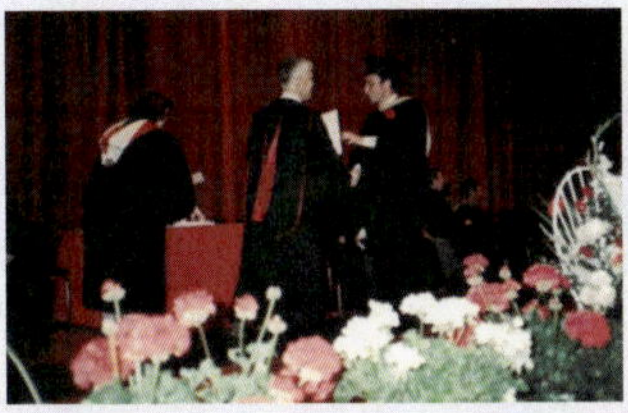

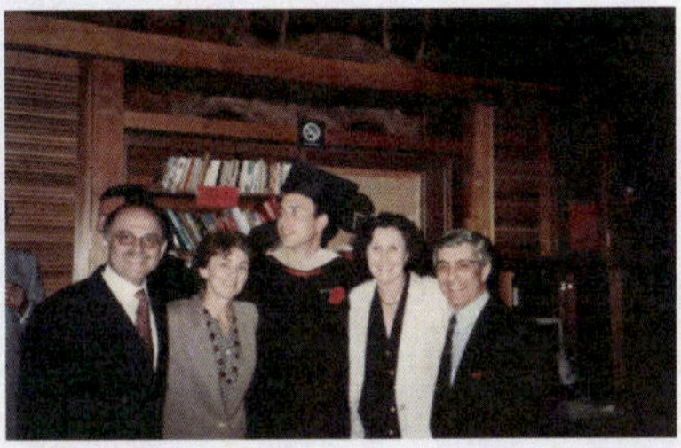

Paul graduated with an MBA from Cornell. We went to his graduation with our close friends Olga and Stan Mermikidis. A great trip.

After graduating with an MBA, Paul worked for several large companies including Credit Suisse, where he created their carbon trading programme. He spoke at many meetings, including two at Davos. I went and heard him speak in Sydney. A very proud father.

Paul did not ask for, or would take any, financial help at all to help pay for his fees or living expenses.

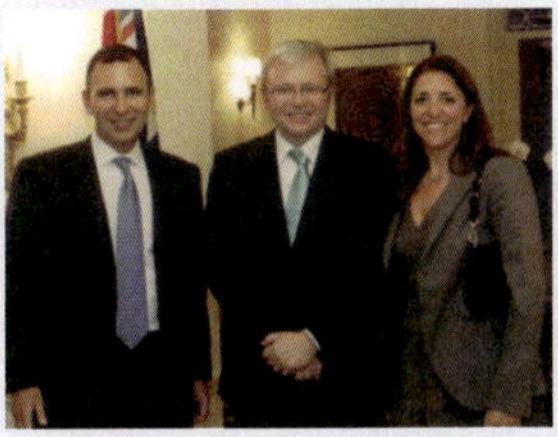

With Australian Prime Minister Kevin Rudd in 2009.

Damon

Damon also went to Scotch College and then did optometry. As there was no optometry school in Perth, he did first year science at the University of Western Australia and then went to the University of New South Wales to complete the optometry course. Barry Collins was the professor of optometry at UNSW and a good friend, so I flew over with Damon to introduce him to Barry. He stayed at Shalom College for the first year and then moved into a flat with some friends for the following two years. To ensure that he did not do without anything, we gave him a credit card and a car so that he could enjoy college life and Sydney. I recall visiting Damon and driving around with him as he pointed out high-end restaurants and told us how good the food was there. I never had this luxury, but we were happy that he had the opportunity.

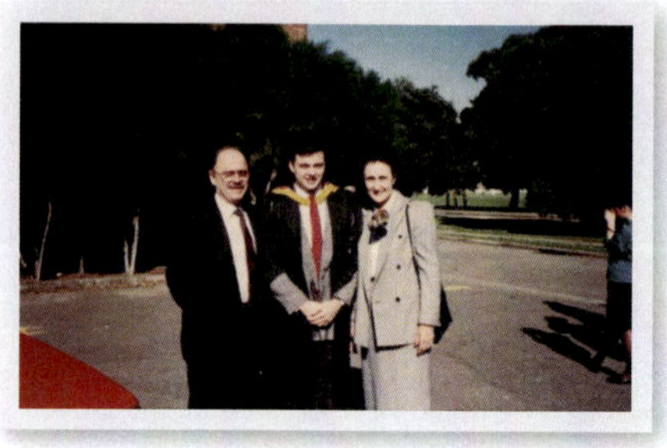

Damon's graduation.

Sasha

Sasha went to PLC and then to the University of Western Australia, studying marketing and public relations, but she was unsettled. She left university and went to a famous cooking school, Ballymaloe, in Ireland. We visited her while she was there, which was very nice. She completed a marketing course when she returned home.

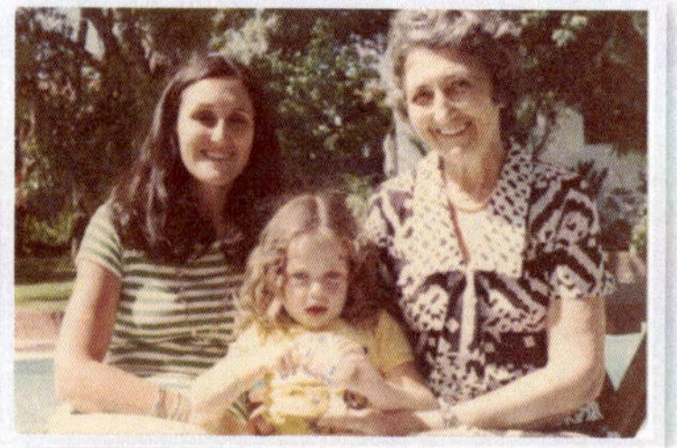

Sasha and Nan Connell. December 1974.

CHAPTER SEVEN

STARTING MY OWN PRACTICE

In December 1971 I started my own practice in a small upstairs office on Kings Park Road. Many old patients supported me and I received regular referrals from doctors.

London and Contact Lens Manufacturing

In May 1972 I returned to London to keep up to date with the latest in contact lenses. I went on a cheap charter flight called Saber Air, stopping in Singapore for a few days. The Singapore Ezekiel family knew what had happened with my father and could not have been nicer and more supportive to me. The charter to London was on an old stretch DC8. It took forever to get to London. We had four stops. The pilot tried not to refuel at a nominated stop before London but then ran so low of fuel he had to land in Germany, without a landing right or a refuelling account. The plane was surrounded by troops and we sat there for hours on the tarmac as they apparently negotiated. Eventually they must have paid for fuel and the plane refuelled and we left Germany. I was pleased to get to London! I stayed in a one-star hotel recommended by a patient off Oxford Street. It was cheap. I had the use of a communal bath and I think I was the only one who used it. One night I came to my room to find it had been ransacked. As I went to report this, an American lady came out of her adjoining room and told me that they had taken her suitcase. Luckily nothing was stolen from me. I had bought Challis a bangle, which fortunately they did not find. After that I put everything in the hotel safe.

I re-visited Moorfields Eye Hospital. Montague Reuben, who was a registrar when I was there in 1967, was now the head of the contact lens department. He always gave me time at my visits and filled me in on the latest contact lens developments. I mentioned to Monty that Joseph Dallos had advised me to make lenses for my patients. Monty said you must, and that he would arrange it. He picked up the phone and called George Nissel (brother-in-law of Dallos, who had left Budapest at the same time). Nissel manufactured contact lens machinery. Monty told him that I would be visiting him the next day and asked him to teach me how to make a lens. He then called Phillip Cowdrey, who with his partner David Clulow owned a laboratory called Contact Lens Manufacturing (later called Sauflon). Monty told Phillip I would be coming to see him after my visit to Nissel, and could he teach me all I needed to know about contact lens manufacturing. Contact Lens Manufacturing were ahead of their time, as they manufactured materials, solutions, machinery and contact lenses. While still a student, David Clulow - although not qualified - advertised contact lenses to patients at a very cheap price. By the time he had graduated he had developed a large practice in a beautifully appointed building in Earls Court over two adjoining buildings. His practice offered a 'lens replacement scheme' where for a fee of (I think) 25 pounds a year, he would replace a patient's lenses at a reasonable price of cost plus 10%. On one of my visits he told me that they had 25,000 patients on the scheme. He was not interested in the price of the lenses, which he made in-house, but with the cash flow he received every year from the lens replacement scheme. Maybe the world's first in-house insurance scheme?

Dallos had always encouraged me to make my own lenses, and not to trust the lenses I was receiving. He said I should research my own new ideas, and that it was not difficult. He also taught me how to research, stressing that it didn't matter what you did, as long as you did it. If things don't turn out just right, stand back and you'll soon see what you are doing wrong.

I called Challis and told her that I would be staying in London a couple of weeks longer to learn how to make contact lenses. Nissel, the contact lens machinery manufacturer owned by George Nissel, was in Hemel Hampstead, some forty-five minutes away by train. At the time, Nissel equipment was the gold standard for contact lens manufacturing equipment. The lathes they supplied were basic lathes that sat on an old kitchen table at Nissel's factory. In between interruptions I sort of learned the manufacturing process. The essential process with lathing a lens with good optics is the correct lathe setup so that the diamond is perfectly centred to the workpiece.

Unless lined up perfectly it was not possible to make lenses with good optics. I never learned how to do this correctly!

The Birth of Gelflex

The equipment I ordered from Nissel arrived some months later and I started the process of learning to make lenses. The equipment was installed in an adjoining room of the practice, with the lathe placed on a basic table. Today's lathes are supplied with a stone top on sturdy metal legs. I remember spending weekends in the lab and usually made just three lenses, none with good optics.

I called the laboratory 'Western Australian Contact Lens Manufacturing', later changing the name to Gelflex Laboratories.

Good contact lens practices in London, like Moorfields Eye Hospital, were using soft lenses of a high water content (55%, 75% and 85%) rather than lenses of a lower water content of 43% material used by Hema in Australia. The soft lens materials that I was trying to make were from high water content (Sauflon 75% and 85%) materials and were unstable and the results not repeatable. They were the worst materials to learn to make soft lenses on!

About a year later I returned to London and was given Peter Bryant's name, who had a contact lens laboratory called Focus. Focus later went bankrupt, as Peter understood that the laws regarding the manufacture of contact lenses were about to be changed, including the manufacture of contact lenses needing to be in a clean room environment. He spent a lot of money on his facility to comply with the expected change in the law but this change never eventuated and he ran out of money.

Peter taught me how to set up the lathe and we made lenses with good optics. Over the years Peter and I swapped ideas and pieces of equipment that we made that were not available for purchase. We purchased a metal lathe and employed a toolmaker at the laboratory. Our toolmaker made crimper devices to make toric lenses, which we gave to Peter. I had no idea that one day he would join us here in Perth.

High Court Writ

On Christmas Eve 1976, just eight months after I started to make lenses, I received a high court writ from the National Patent Development Corporation (NPDC) advising that they owned patents to manufacture soft contact lenses in a dry form and then hydrate them in a solution to form a soft lens, and that I was infringing their patent. Four companies received the writ. Two were importers who stopped importing. The third was Penryn Thomas's Corneal Lens Corporation, the largest contact lens laboratory in Australia, which NPDC took over and later became Hydron. I understand that Penryn did not do well and NPDC essentially just acquired the laboratory. This left just me, with a wife, three small children and an overdraft, to defend the writ.

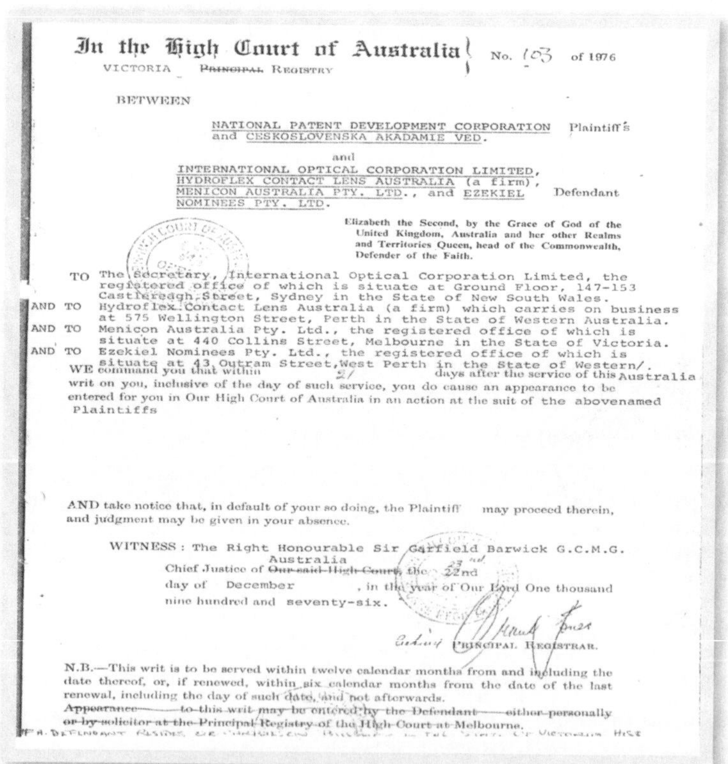

In the High Court of Australia No. 103 of 1976
VICTORIA ~~Principal~~ Registry

BETWEEN

NATIONAL PATENT DEVELOPMENT CORPORATION and CESKOSLOVENSKA AKADAMIE VED. Plaintiffs

and

INTERNATIONAL OPTICAL CORPORATION LIMITED, HYDROFLEX CONTACT LENS AUSTRALIA (a firm), MENICON AUSTRALIA PTY. LTD., and EZEKIEL NOMINEES PTY. LTD. Defendant

Elizabeth the Second, by the Grace of God of the United Kingdom, Australia and her other Realms and Territories Queen, head of the Commonwealth, Defender of the Faith.

TO The Secretary, International Optical Corporation Limited, the registered office of which is situate at Ground Floor, 147-153 Castlereagh Street, Sydney in the State of New South Wales.
AND TO Hydroflex Contact Lens Australia (a firm) which carries on business at 575 Wellington Street, Perth in the State of Western Australia.
AND TO Menicon Australia Pty. Ltd., the registered office of which is situate at 440 Collins Street, Melbourne in the State of Victoria.
AND TO Ezekiel Nominees Pty. Ltd., the registered office of which is situate at 43 Outram Street, West Perth in the State of Western Australia.

WE command you that within 21 days after the service of this writ on you, inclusive of the day of such service, you do cause an appearance to be entered for you in Our High Court of Australia in an action at the suit of the abovenamed Plaintiffs

AND take notice that, in default of your so doing, the Plaintiff may proceed therein, and judgment may be given in your absence.

WITNESS: The Right Honourable Sir Garfield Barwick G.C.M.G. Chief Justice of ~~Our said High Court~~ Australia, the 22nd day of December, in the year of Our Lord One thousand nine hundred and seventy-six.

Acting PRINCIPAL REGISTRAR.

N.B.—This writ is to be served within twelve calendar months from and including the date thereof, or, if renewed, within six calendar months from the date of the last renewal, including the day of such date, and not afterwards.
~~Appearance to this writ may be entered by the Defendant either personally or by solicitor at the Principal Registry of the High Court at Melbourne.~~

A high court writ must be replied to within thirty days, and the reply to the high court must be by a Queens Counsel, with the assistance of an Assistant Queens Council, and a patent attorney instructed by a lawyer. None knew anything about contact lenses!

John Lemonis, my Perth lawyer, advised the best patent attorney was in Melbourne, so I travelled there. I remember sitting in the book-lined office of a Queens Council with an Assistant Queens Council, a patent attorney and a lawyer, thinking, "What am I - a simple optometrist trying to make contact lenses for my patients - doing here?"

Many overseas people were a great help in supplying details of published papers describing 'prior art' of the infringement claims stated. I think laboratories were concerned that if this case was lost it would create a patent problem for them and they would be sued and perhaps lose their businesses.

Our legal team replied to the high court. Nothing further was heard for some time so my legal team advised me they were closing the file. It was my introduction to the way large companies protect their market by threatening and forcing potential competitors away. They partly succeeded.

Outram Street

After eighteen months in Kings Park Road I was running out of space and not happy being in a rented place. Challis saw an advertisement for a property for sale in Outram Street in West Perth. The overseas owner became sick and thought he was going to die, so put the property on the market. He wanted $62,000. I offered him $58,000 and bought it. I borrowed all the money and moved over Christmas by myself, pushing the equipment on a trolley over several blocks to the new premises. The Muscular Dystrophy Association tenanted two back rooms, which helped pay the mortgage. The lab was placed in the front room of the building, which later became the practice waiting room. The practice grew and I saw interesting patients who helped me develop lenses that allowed them to achieve good vision.

I also had several experiences that made the practice interesting and worthwhile.

When the world cricket series came to Australia, Madgid Khan, a prominent Pakistani cricketer, made centuries in all his matches around the country. While in Adelaide, he lost a contact lens. When the team came to Perth he consulted me and we made him a pair of contact lenses. He then made two ducks. I saw him after the match and apologised profusely but he said it was the end of the tour and he was tired. The lenses were fine. Maybe I did my part?

In 1978, as a result of stress from the high court writ, I ended up in hospital with a suspected heart problem. It turned out to be just stress related exhaustion. The stay in hospital was good as it made me realise I was trying to do more than I could do and should get some help in the busy practice. I advertised and employed an optometrist. The tenant left and we made another consulting room.

I also realised that it was not ideal to have the lab in the practice. I thought I could do things better than the technicians, but I was only getting in the way. While the lab was in Outram Street I would go in early each morning and check the lenses we made the previous day; usually only about eighteen lenses in the day.

Soon after my stay in hospital we saw an advertisement for a building for sale several blocks away in Mayfair Street, West Perth. My doctor told me to take it easy and not to have any excitement so I asked a good friend, Rodney Cohen, to come with me to the auction. We bought the building and moved the lab there. Again, we borrowed the full amount of $68,000.

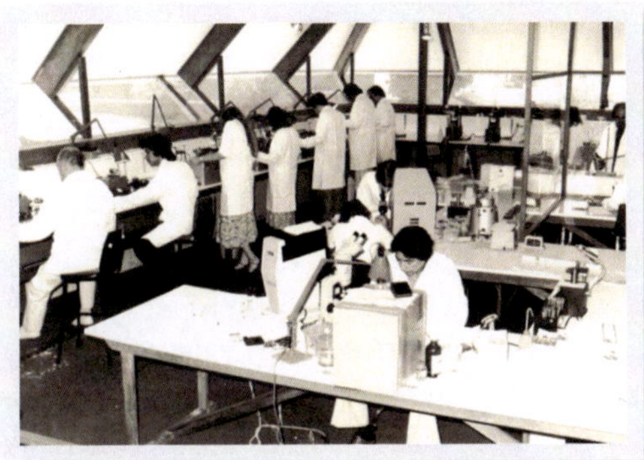

Mayfair Street laboratory.

The lab grew slowly. We made several attempts with eastern states representatives and even hired a serviced room in Sydney with an optometrist as a representative, but none were successful. We received no support from local optometrists.

I was aware that I did not have anyone experienced in the laboratory in contact lens manufacturing. I advertised overseas and managed to recruit several technicians but not one turned out to be good technicians and only brought their personal problems with them!

We had a problem making quality reproducible lenses as the basic Nissel lathes required final lens hand edge finishing by a technician. We purchased Swiss Gfeller lathes that allowed better quality lenses to be made. The lathes were important when we made the IOGEL interocular lenses as the lens design was created on a template, allowing reproduceable intraocular lenses to be made.

In 1988 I saw an advertisement in a journal from DAC, a US company in Santa Barbara, advertising computerised lathes. I visited them shortly afterwards and bought two four-axis lathes and a mill. I think I was one of the first to purchase a lathe from DAC. They are now one of the premier contact lens lathe manufacturers in the world.

Barry Connell

Barry is Challis's brother. I knew him before I met Challis in 1957; when Challis and I were on the *Gorgon* on our way to Singapore on our honeymoon, the ship called into Geraldton. I saw Barry and called out to him, much to Challis's surprise!

Barry later joined Gelflex and subsequently became laboratory manager. I remember taking him with me to London so he could get some exposure of contact lens manufacturing. On the day we arrived we were invited by a supplier for dinner. Barry excused himself as he said he was tired, so I went alone. I returned later that night to find no Barry. He arrived back very much later. Where had he been? As we were free the following night Barry suggested we go to a club. He took me to a strip club, where on arrival he was greeted with "Hello Barry!" Barry soon realised the strip club was not my scene, so we didn't stay long and went to a pub instead. Again we were greeted with "Hello Barry!" Barry was a loveable character who sadly died at a young age from cancer. We all miss him.

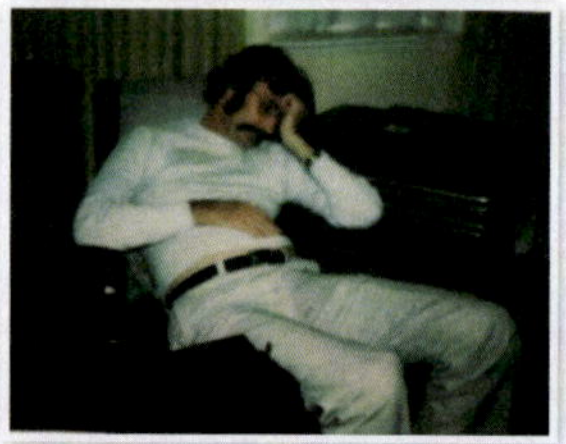

Barry working next day in London.

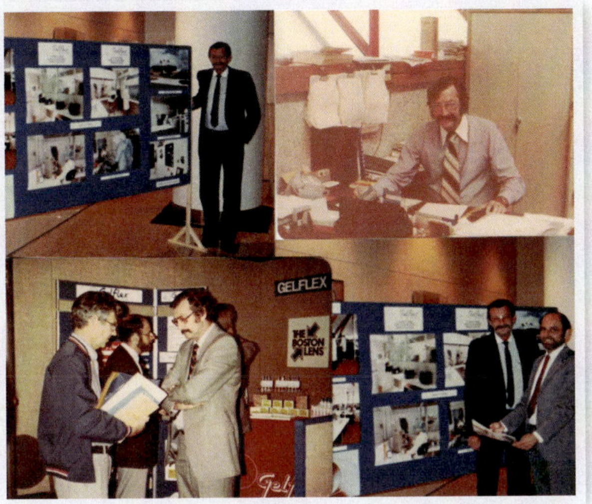

Barry manning stands at meetings.

Grant Connell

Barry's son Grant joined Gelflex some years later. He was an excellent addition to the laboratory and was a loyal, hardworking and trustworthy employee.

When the laboratory was acquired it moved to larger premises and Grant was responsible in designing the layout of the laboratory. Gelflex subsequently bought a Melbourne custom lab and sent Grant to Melbourne to get the lab up to the standard of a contact lens laboratory. I subsequently learned that the Melbourne laboratory was to be closed and all custom lens work to be made in Perth. Such a shame as Grant was an important person in the laboratory with great knowledge of contact lenses. Gelflex was the loser!

IOGEL

In 1983 I gave a lecture at the laboratory to a group of ophthalmology registrars on contact lenses. After the lecture Graham Barrett, one of the registrars, stayed behind and asked if I could make an Intra Ocular Lens (IOL) from Hema for him. I asked Graham how many he needed. He replied if it worked, many millions. He gave me a complex design. We could not make it accurately with the lathes we then had, so the design was modified and we made IOL with Hema material. We called it the IOGEL lens.

I later learned from Graham that he had heard a lecture by a Doctor Epstein, a South African ophthalmologist, who described an IOL made from Hema. Epstein had the idea of a soft IOL made from a hydrogel material but never had one lens made or implanted. I applied for and paid for all patents received for the lens design incorporating the use of the Hema material to manufacture an IOL. Graham then did not want me to have any ongoing interest in the project, so I refused to do any more with the lens unless I had a share of the project. He reluctantly agreed and we shared any proceeds from the project.

Graham was an ophthalmology registrar (studying to become an ophthalmologist) and implanted more than thirty lenses under the supervision of ophthalmologist Ian Stewart at Royal Perth Hospital. The results were all good. But what were we going to do with the lens?

Alcon

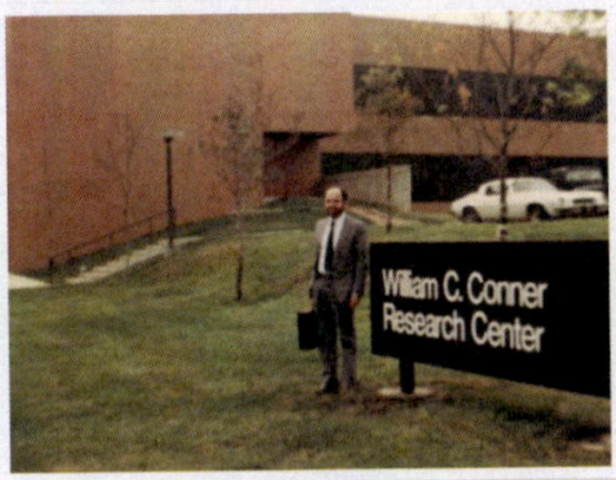

Alcon.

I did some research and found that Alcon, a part of Nestle, the world's largest ophthalmic company, did not have an IOL lens. I made one phone call and obtained the name and direct phone number of Tim Sear, the vice president of Alcon in Fort Worth, Texas. There is a fourteen-hour time difference between Perth and Fort Worth. I remember sitting up in bed late at night in my pyjamas and calling Tim Sear. "You do not know me, but this is what we have developed." I subsequently learned the person who gave me Tim's number had called him and informed him on the reason for my call. The timing was right. Alcon were looking to get into the IOL market.

I spent several hours over the following nights on calls with personnel at Alcon, answering their questions. They asked me to go to Fort Worth, but I suggested it best for them to send an ophthalmologist who was familiar with IOLs to come to Perth and we would show him the result of implanted lenses. If they were happy and wanted to proceed with an arrangement, then I would come to Fort Worth.

Within the week they had ophthalmologist Richard Keats, a prominent high-profile authority of intraocular lenses, in Perth. Graham Barrett showed him patients implanted with the lens and he was impressed. I was then asked to purchase a ticket to Fort Worth, for which they would reimburse me. I purchased a first class ticket - they later told me they only travel business class, not first class!

When my brother Eric had left Perth to live in Israel, he had asked me to find a tenant for his house in Dalkeith. We advertised and Peter and Barbara Eastwood replied and rented the house. They had only just arrived from South Africa and did not know anyone, so we invited them and their two children to spend Christmas with us. We became good friends. Peter was a Harvard graduate and subsequently went to live in Ohio, USA. I called and asked him to come to Fort Worth and help me with the negotiations. He flew down to Fort Worth and we met at Dallas Fort Worth airport.

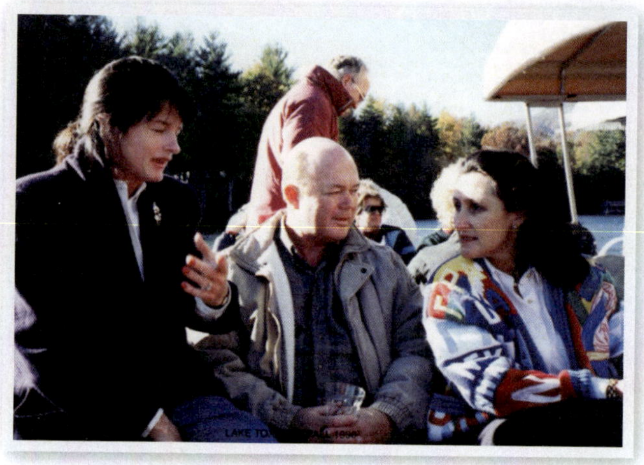

Barbara and Peter Eastwood with Challis at a golf course in the USA.

We were picked up in a stretch limo from the airport and taken to meet Tim Sear, along with Alcon patent attorneys, lawyers and engineers. I told them that Peter was a business friend and would help me with negotiating a potential arrangement. I was shown around their research facility, which was amazing, while they discussed a possible deal with Peter. On my return I was told that they had made an offer to Peter. He and I were then placed in a room and told not to hurry. Peter told me they offered $100,000. I said no. I think it was worth more. Peter agreed and suggested we should leave and he would get his lawyer in Ohio, who was a great negotiator, to negotiate for me.

Within a few minutes the door flew open and Tim Sear and his group came into the room. I told them what they offered was not acceptable. They doubled it. Peter's eyes lit up. I again said no. I thought the lens was worth more and needed to take further advice. We were picked up in a limo when we arrived, but were returned to the airport in a van! We flew to Peter's home in Ohio.

Peter told me his lawyer Mel Schottenstein, a great negotiator, was booked out for several weeks but would give me ten minutes. We met with Mel and he gave me over an hour. At one stage his secretary called to say that group X were in to see him. He told her to put them in the Y room and serve them lunch.

He never asked what we had, but asked who the big IOL players were. I gave him their names and it appeared that he was a director on boards with all the major companies mentioned. He called them and asked the market size for the lens and what it was worth. He then asked me who my patent attorney was. I told him Kelvin Lord. "Let's get him on the phone," he said. I told him it was four am in Perth. "Good. He will probably be home."

Then he told me I had to stay at least two weeks, as he needed time to negotiate. I called Challis and told her I needed to stay away longer.

All the time I was in Ohio waiting for Mel Schottenstein to call me to come to his office, Graham was calling and giving me a hard time telling me that I should hurry up and do a more thorough job. Just what I needed!

But Mel had played the game well. I remember the final day he finalised the negotiations with Alcon. They were in Fort Worth; we were in Ohio. He had his feet on his desk which had nothing on it apart from a speaker phone (a lawyer with no paper on his desk?) and spoke to them from one of many speaker phones in the room. At one stage he asked a basic question he had asked earlier and left the room for about ten minutes while the Alcon people went over it all again. A very interesting experience for me.

Mel made a good deal in that we were to receive some money up front, plus make the first 5,000 lenses at a good price. It even included Alcon paying for the first $20,000 of Mel's legal fees.

Alcon started to sell the IOGEL (later called Hydrosoft) but never really got the lens to market. They subsequently bought several IOL laboratories that were using better materials than Hema and effectively warehoused our lens until they had their own equivalent lens available in a different material. Apart from our contract to make the first 25,000 lenses, the expected royalties did not materialise, but the upfront money did allow me to finance the building of the solutions laboratory.

To be fair to Alcon, one of the IOL laboratories they purchased had a new and better material than the Hema we used so understandably they moved to use this material for their IOL lenses.

One great benefit of working with Alcon was they sent their Quality Assurance personnel to Perth to supervise the packaging and helped us put together all the necessary paperwork to get Food and Drug Association (FDA) approval for implantable lenses.

Alcon supplied the vials for lens packaging and sent their QA person to ensure the first lens packaging was done correctly. The final lens packaging involved the lens being placed in a solution in a specially designed vial and sterilised by autoclave. After the first autoclaving the lenses turned brown. The vial screw caps supplied by Alcon included a cork seal, which caused the lenses to discolour. New vials with a crimp seal were made and supplied for the final lens packaging. This delayed our supply of lenses to Alcon and their payments to us that I depended on to finance the solution laboratory. Paul and I visited Alcon in Fort Worth and explained to the company's president Schmolmyer and vice president Tim Sear that our cash flow problem was due to the faulty vials supplied. They agreed to payments in advance to help with our cash flow. Very decent - even though the delay was their fault.

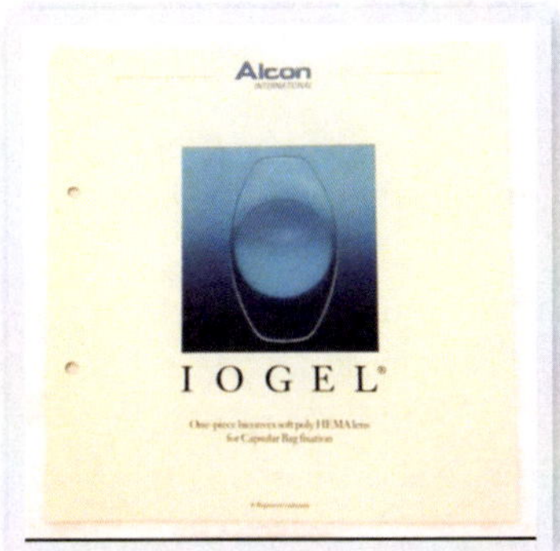

Marketing material for the IOGEL lens.

In August 1992 Alcon advised they had decided not to further pursue the IOGEL lens. We just had to put it down to experience. One thing we have learned from this is that we must do our own marketing. We would try to do this with the translating bifocal lens.

CHAPTER EIGHT
GELFLEX LABORATORIES

Gelflex Pharmaceutical Laboratory

Our Melbourne representative, Duncan Stevens, saw an opening to make normal saline used to sterilise soft contact lenses. We rented a small unit in Dandenong, an outer suburb of Melbourne, purchased second-hand equipment and made saline. The saline was manually bottled and sent to a carpet manufacturer to be gamma sterilised. This resulted in us having a good share of the Australian contact lens saline market.

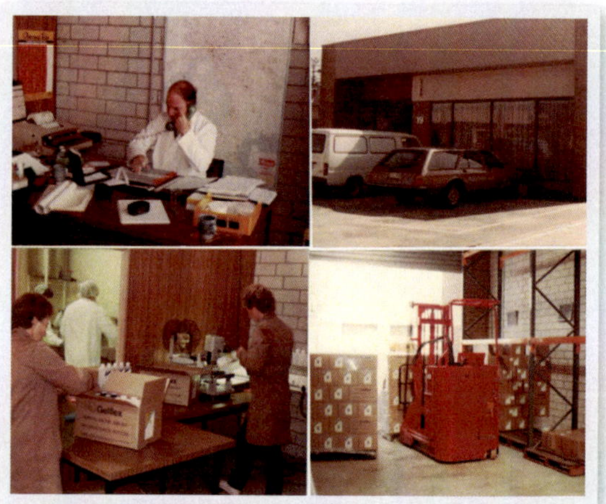

Initial solution laboratory.

If it was easy to make saline, so why not make intravenous solutions?

In February 1981 we bought a large block of land in Healy Road, Dandenong, and built a solutions laboratory. I went to Interpack, a packaging trade show in Germany. In the pharmaceutical pavilion was displayed an automatic bottle-making and filling machine company called Rommelag that supplied machinery that, in a thirty-second cycle, blew four bottles, filled and sealed them with solution ready for sterilisation. I ordered a Rommelag unit.

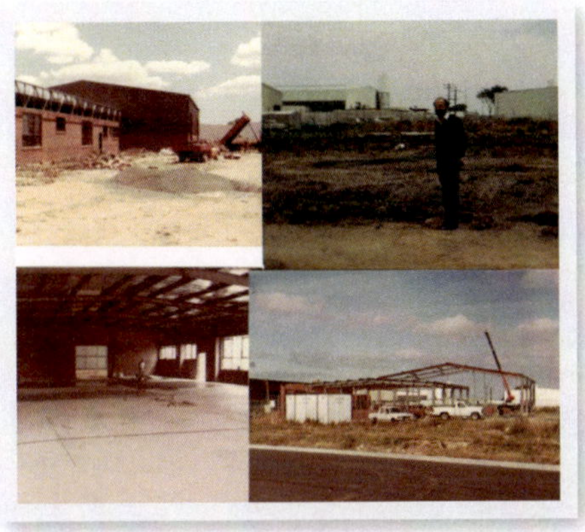

Site of solution laboratory building.

Meanwhile, a pharmaceutical laboratory in Perth told the government that there were no Rommelag machines in Australia, so the Western Australian government purchased a Rommelag machine for them!

We already had one that we had financed ourselves with no help – at a time when bank rates were 24%! I called the government guy to tell him this and he said he hadn't known, and asked me to please not make it public. I never learned how to work the system. That Perth lab was later sold to multinational Pfizer for millions.

I was given the name of a small laboratory in Ireland that was producing the solutions we were interested in making. I visited it and for a fee was provided with details of where to purchase the equipment needed, such as a water still and an autoclave, and the formulas to get started.

On their recommendation, I purchased an autoclave manufactured in Brisbane by a Swedish company. The unit was a lemon and continually broke down. Duncan Stevens later sourced a replacement autoclave from an Austrian company and he and I went to Austria and bought a very good computer-controlled autoclave.

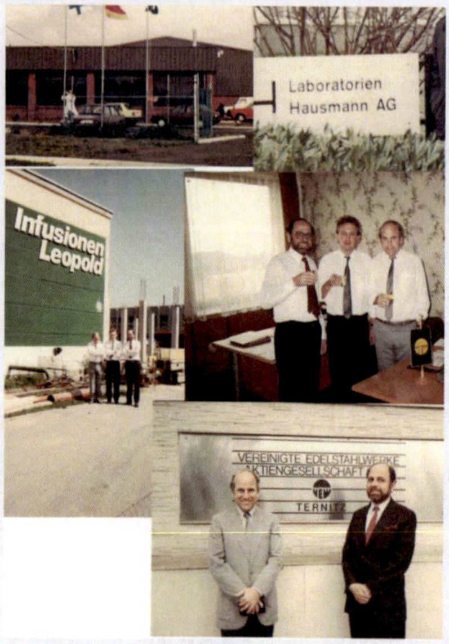

Visiting the Austrian autoclave company with Duncan Stevens.

Having the new autoclave meant we had to expand the area of the laboratory. We learned from our earlier mistake of making the packaging area too small, so we added a large packaging and larger warehouse area.

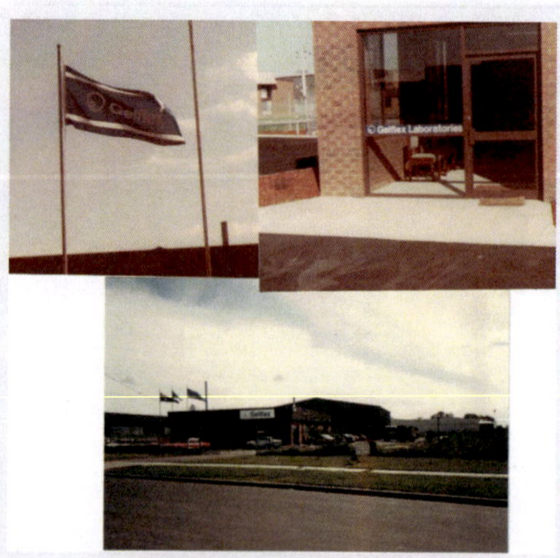

New Gelflex Solution Laboratory incorporating the new autoclave and larger warehouse area.

Hospitals in Australia wanted Intra Venous (IV) solutions in bags, but the Rommelag filled solutions in bottles. The problem with bottles for hospitals was their disposal after use. Bags are much easier to dispose of. So we made our own machine to make IV bags. We sourced the material from the Netherlands, but our method of manufacture and filling was very labour intensive. I again went to the Interpack trade show in Germany and sourced a fully automated system where the bag was made and filled in one process.

We were competing with Baxter Travenol, a large multinational company who controlled the Australian IV market. Once we started offering sterile IV solutions in a bag form, Travenol halved the price of their IV solutions to hospitals. On one occasion we received a large order from the Royal Melbourne Hospital only for it to be cancelled by the time our representative returned to the laboratory. On asking them why the order was cancelled, the hospital told us that if they followed through with the order with Gelflex, Travenol would increase the cost of all the other supplies they brought from them, and the forklift given to the hospital by Travenol would have to be given back.

If I knew then what I know now, I would have reported them to the ACCC and we maybe would have survived. As it was, with 24% interest rates it was very difficult. I should also have looked for outside funding. At the Small Business Award ceremony, when Gelflex won a major award, many senior people from businesses who were interested in investing with us gave me their business cards. I always remember my father saying not to have a business partner, so I took his advice and did not follow any up. In hindsight this was a big mistake. I should have taken in a partner, as with some external cash input the solutions lab would have survived and prospered. It was a good project but too large for our small company with a limited cash flow. We contract manufactured a product at the time to a company called Gambro. They wanted to purchase the lab, so we sold it to them. Had they not purchased the lab I would probably have gone bankrupt.

The other problem was the ANZ bank. The man responsible for my account would call almost every day to see how I was getting on. Just pressure-pressure-pressure. I had cashed in all my super to survive.

State and National Small Business Award

In 1985 Gelflex Laboratories won the state and national Small Business Award.

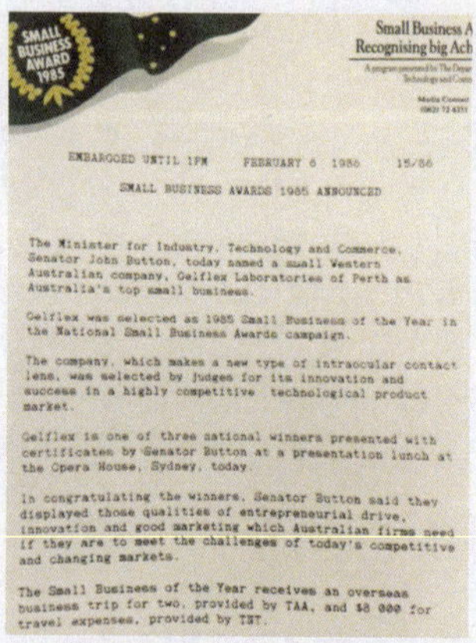

SMALL BUSINESS AWARD 1985

Small Business A
Recognising big Ach

EMBARGOED UNTIL 1PM FEBRUARY 6 1986 15/86

SMALL BUSINESS AWARDS 1985 ANNOUNCED

The Minister for Industry, Technology and Commerce, Senator John Button, today named a small Western Australian company, Gelflex Laboratories of Perth as Australia's top small business.

Gelflex was selected as 1985 Small Business of the Year in the National Small Business Awards campaign.

The company, which makes a new type of intraocular contact lens, was selected by judges for its innovation and success in a highly competitive technological product market.

Gelflex is one of three national winners presented with certificates by Senator Button at a presentation lunch at the Opera House, Sydney, today.

In congratulating the winners, Senator Button said they displayed those qualities of entrepreneurial drive, innovation and good marketing which Australian firms need if they are to meet the challenges of today's competitive and changing markets.

The Small Business of the Year receives an overseas business trip for two, provided by TAA, and $8 000 for travel expenses, provided by TNT.

The national final was at luncheon held at the Sydney Opera House, and the award was presented to me by the Federal Minister of Industry and Commerce, John Dutton. It was a well-attended occasion with reports on our win in papers and business magazines, including the *Business Review*. This story is in the Appendix.

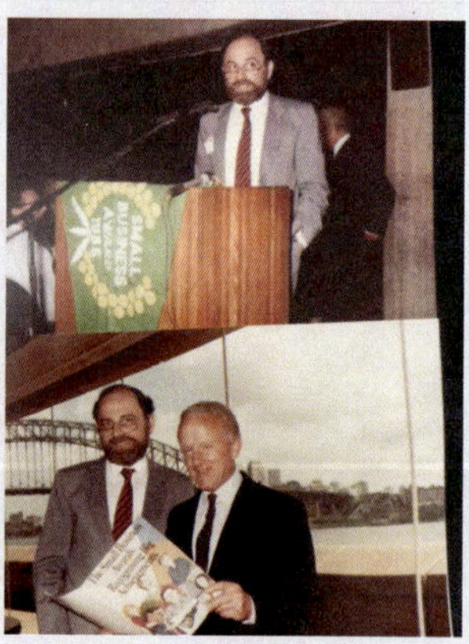

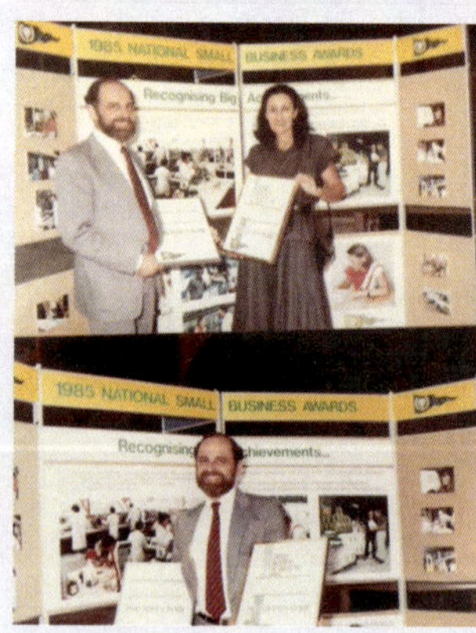

With the Federal Minister for Industry, Senator John Button

CHAPTER NINE

INTERNATIONAL SOCIETY OF CONTACT LENS SPECIALISTS

The ISCLS

In 1983 a US optometrist friend, Mel Remba, suggested that I might like to attend a meeting of the International Society of Contact Lens Specialists (ISCLS). This is an invited-only group with about sixty-five members. Challis and I attended the meeting in Versailles, which was organised by Pierre Rocher, who I knew when we were on our travels around Europe in Paris in 1963 and who I had purchased lens modification equipment from. It was a fantastic meeting. Many contact lenses legends were there. I read a paper on the gas permeable scleral lenses and showed a video I had made titled 'A Practitioners Guide to Fitting Gas Permeable Scleral Lenses'.

After reading two papers at ISCLS meetings you may be invited to join. They also check on one's wife to ensure that she was a compatible fit with the group. I became a member and in 2003, I received the Hershel medal from the ISCLS. A great honour. In 2012, I became an Honorary Life Member. Some years later I introduced Damon to ISCLS. He became a member and subsequently became the president of the society.

ISCLS meetings we attended included Berlin, Washington, England, Buenos Aires, Berlin, Belfast and Charleston USA. All were wonderful and we both enjoyed the meetings and the company.

Post-congress travels organised by the meeting's hosts were special and allowed us to see parts of countries we would never have otherwise gone to. Afternoon tea at Versailles and an opera in Dresden were just some of the wonderful experiences we had.

In 1983 I also became a member of the American Academy of Optometry. In 1984 I received a letter from Roger Kame, President of the Academy, asking if I would present a paper to them on scleral lenses. The Academy has a higher degree in contact lenses than a Diploma in Contact Lenses. This involves writing eight patient case histories followed by an oral and written exam. One of the eight sections was to write a case history on a specialist lens. I described my fitting of scleral lenses and included the paper I read at the annual meeting of the British Contact Lens Association (BCLA), and published by the BCLA. My case reports were not accepted, as the examiner responded by asking if I had ever even fitted a scleral lens (!).

I did not continue with the Diploma process any further.

Donald Korb

I was first introduced to Donald Korb by prominent South African optometrist Grant Jenkins. Our laboratory had been using high water content blanks sourced from Sauflon to manufacture soft lenses. A laboratory was established in Los Angeles by Sauflon for a group of furniture manufacturing investors as Sauflon USA, using Sauflon high water content material to manufacture extended lens wear lenses for a large potential market. They were having trouble making the lenses and asked me to visit the US facility to report on the process and the quality of the lenses made. I met Grant on the visit to the laboratory as he also was asked to advise on the US lab's manufacturing. Our audit of the laboratory was not positive and it closed. As we were both going to the BCLA meeting in London, Grant and I decided to travel together. Grant suggested that we stop over in Boston and catch up with a friend of his, Donald Korb. Donald is the most innovative and clever optometrist I have ever met. He designed an early soft lens and is the world's expert on dry eyes. He is also the most loveable, interesting character and we became good friends.

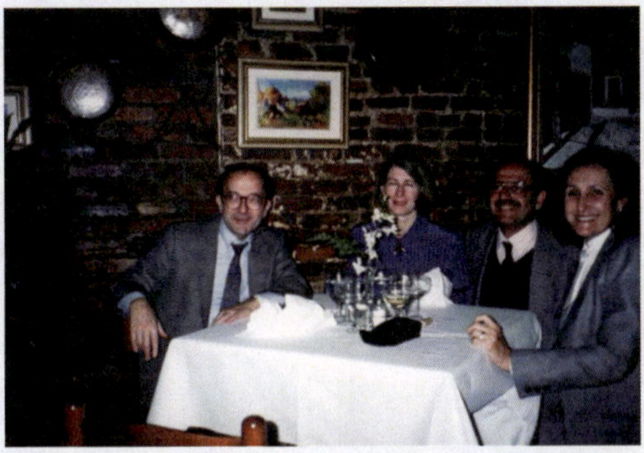

With Donald and Joan in Boston.

Donald and his wife Joan visited Perth some years later and stayed with us. At the visit I told Donald about how I had presented a paper and showed a video on gas permeable scleral lenses at the meeting of the ISCLS, and how a doctor asked if I had ever fitted a lens. I asked Donald how he would have handled this. He said he would have replied, "That's a great question!" and then gone on to say whatever he wanted to say, not answering the question.

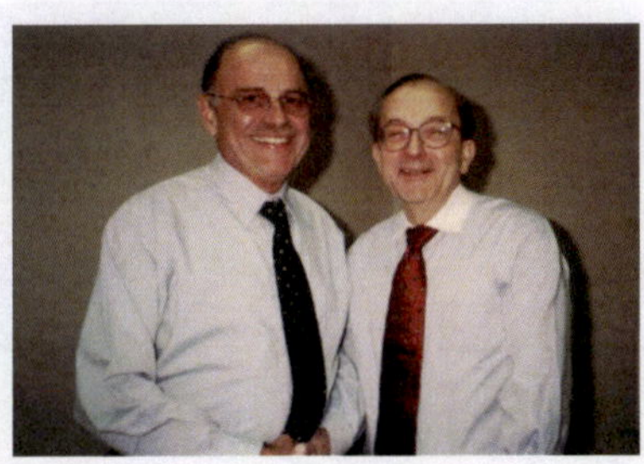

While Donald was in Perth, I arranged for him to speak at a meeting of the local contact lens society. When someone asked him a question he looked at me and said, "That's a great question!" and then spoke about something quite different. He became a close friend and we stayed with them in Boston on several occasions. One of the world's true loveable characters. Donald told of his returning home after an interstate visit to find an unknown person in the kitchen who asked him if he was a guest. They told him where the goodies were and suggested he check out a bed before they were all taken!

When an Expert is Not a Specialist

In 1985 I fitted a scleral lens for a keratoconus patient who lived in the north of the state. The government had a scheme where people who lived in remote areas could receive assistance to come to Perth for treatment. The patient applied for financial assistance but was refused. He appealed to the tribunal but was refused again, as although I was seen as a specialist in contact lenses, I was not referred by a doctor, so was not recognised as specialist. There was a lot of publicity on the decision. This is one article.

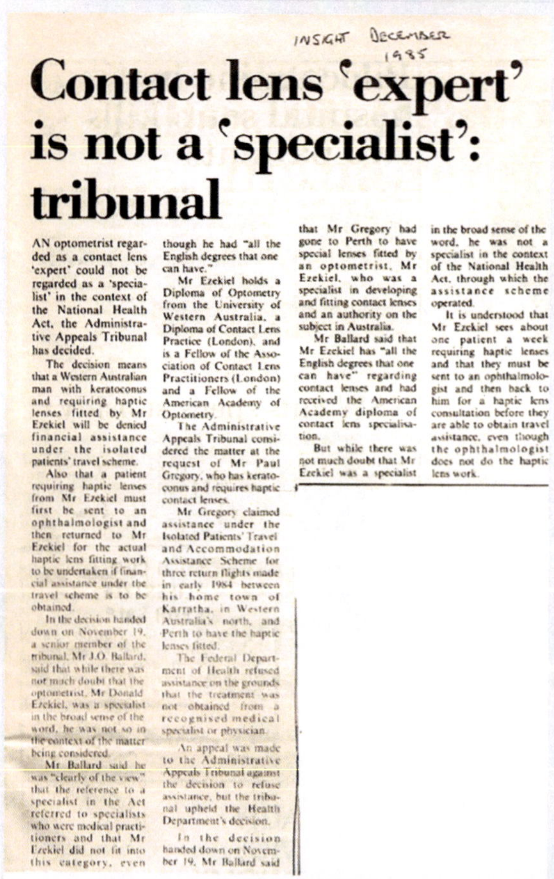

INSIGHT DECEMBER 1985

Contact lens 'expert' is not a 'specialist': tribunal

AN optometrist regarded as a contact lens 'expert' could not be regarded as a 'specialist' in the context of the National Health Act, the Administrative Appeals Tribunal has decided.

The decision means that a Western Australian man with keratoconus and requiring haptic lenses fitted by Mr Ezekiel will be denied financial assistance under the isolated patients' travel scheme.

Also that a patient requiring haptic lenses from Mr Ezekiel must first be sent to an ophthalmologist and then returned to Mr Ezekiel for the actual haptic lens fitting work to be undertaken if financial assistance under the travel scheme is to be obtained.

In the decision handed down on November 19, a senior member of the tribunal, Mr J.O. Ballard, said that while there was not much doubt that the optometrist, Mr Donald Ezekiel, was a specialist in the broad sense of the word, he was not so in the context of the matter being considered.

Mr Ballard said he was "clearly of the view" that the reference to a specialist in the Act referred to specialists who were medical practitioners and that Mr Ezekiel did not fit into this category, even though he had "all the English degrees that one can have."

Mr Ezekiel holds a Diploma of Optometry from the University of Western Australia, a Diploma of Contact Lens Practice (London), and is a Fellow of the Association of Contact Lens Practitioners (London) and a Fellow of the American Academy of Optometry.

The Administrative Appeals Tribunal considered the matter at the request of Mr Paul Gregory, who has keratoconus and requires haptic contact lenses.

Mr Gregory claimed assistance under the Isolated Patients' Travel and Accommodation Assistance Scheme for three return flights made in early 1984 between his home town of Karratha, in Western Australia's north, and Perth to have the haptic lenses fitted.

The Federal Department of Health refused assistance on the grounds that the treatment was not obtained from a recognised medical specialist or physician.

An appeal was made to the Administrative Appeals Tribunal against the decision to refuse assistance, but the tribunal upheld the Health Department's decision.

In the decision handed down on November 19, Mr Ballard said that Mr Gregory had gone to Perth to have special lenses fitted by an optometrist, Mr Ezekiel, who was a specialist in developing and fitting contact lenses and an authority on the subject in Australia.

Mr Ballard said that Mr Ezekiel has "all the English degrees that one can have" regarding contact lenses and had received the American Academy diploma of contact lens specialisation.

But while there was not much doubt that Mr Ezekiel was a specialist in the broad sense of the word, he was not a specialist in the context of the National Health Act, through which the assistance scheme operated.

It is understood that Mr Ezekiel sees about one patient a week requiring haptic lenses and that they must be sent to an ophthalmologist and then back to him for a haptic lens consultation before they are able to obtain travel assistance, even though the ophthalmologist does not do the haptic lens work.

CHAPTER TEN

BREAKING INTO THE USA

Scioptic

Sometime around 1990 a man called Gene Zamba visited our laboratory. He asked why we did not sell lenses in the USA. I told him that the FDA approval was too hard for a little guy like me. He told me it was not difficult and he would do it for a small fee. He applied for, and we received, FDA approval.

Gene introduced us to a David Amar as someone who would market the lenses in the USA. Amar set up a company called Scioptic and began to import our lenses. Initially our lens design was too thick for the USA market, so we altered the design and they began to sell.

David arranged meetings and I went to the USA and spent three days lecturing on lenses. As in Australia, the knowledge in the USA on specialist contact lenses was minimal.

Hutton Street Laboratory

It looked like the USA market was going to be good for us, as Zamba told me that he could sell everything we made! (I never learn, I believe everyone!). As the Mayfair Street building was not really suitable for a laboratory (every time we bought a new lathe, we had to take the roof off to get the lathe into the first floor) and we were running out of space, I looked around for a larger building for the laboratory.

A building in Hutton Street, Osborne Park came up. It was rented by the National Bank for one of their computer networks but had not been used for over a year. There was a year remaining in their lease and the owner wanted $1.1 million for the building. We bought it for $960,000, moved the laboratory there and built a large clean room, in expectation of continuing IOGEL orders from Alcon, along with the orders from Scioptic.

We sold Mayfair Street but still needed to borrow money from the bank. The ANZ was giving me a really hard time, so I told them that after 20-odd years with them I was going to move. A patient recommended the St. George Bank. They gave me a very much better deal than the ANZ with better rates and more borrowings.

As we were getting busier I needed to get someone to run the lab production. I called Peter Bryant in London. I knew that Peter had lost his lab (Focus) in the UK and was working for several lens material and diamond suppliers. He had visited Perth some four years earlier when he had a job with contact lens equipment supplier, City Crown. I timed it well and Peter came and joined the lab.

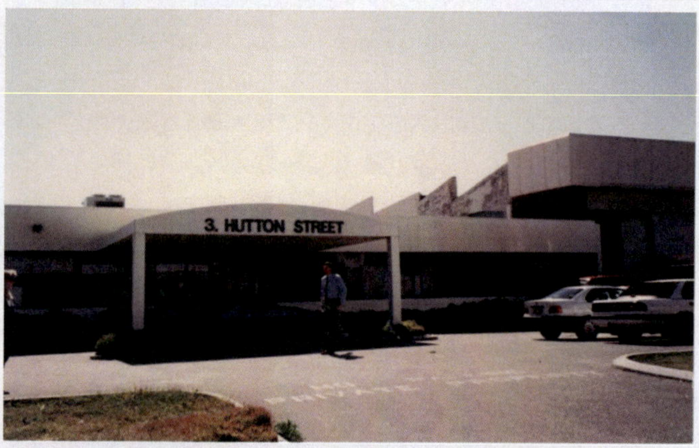

Hutton Street building.

Celflex USA

David Amar's company, Scioptic, was still purchasing lenses to sell in the USA. He was paying his bills regularly but later stopped paying on the 30-day account we had agreed to. Amar arranged for me to meet with doctors wherever I was lecturing around the USA. One time, he booked a meeting for the wrong month, and an account for about $175,000 was sent to Scioptic for the missed meeting. To avoid paying the account, he applied for Chapter 11 bankruptcy and changed the company name to Scioptic International. Because of this he could not borrow money, so in effect we became his banker! He owed us a lot of money. Screwed again.

John Hagendorf was running the US office in Danbury, about an hour out of New York. John was a professional golfer playing on the second circuit. He told me how difficult it was for a second-tier golfer to get to tournaments, sharing a car with a group of four, all sharing a single motel room, often sleeping in the bath and only getting money if they played well. John is a really nice person, so I called him and told him that we were planning to stop supplying Amar and would be opening our own office, and would he like to join us. He was shocked but pleased.

I travelled to New York. Paul and I went to Danbury in Connecticut and looked for office space. Our lawyers served a writ on Amar for the money he owed us and we started fresh, with John Hagendorf marketing directly to the doctors.

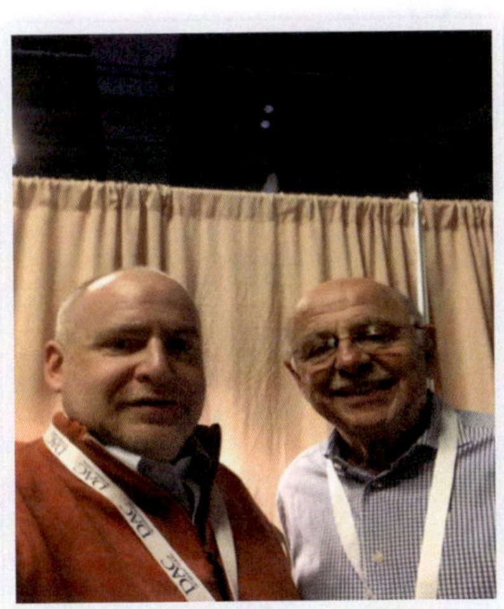

John Hagendorf, Manager US Office.

AM Award

In January 1999, I was a made a Member of the Order of Australia (AM) for my work with contact lenses, and especially with the scleral lens. The presentation was held in Government House. Challis, Damon and Sasha came to the presentation and were proud of me. It was very nice.

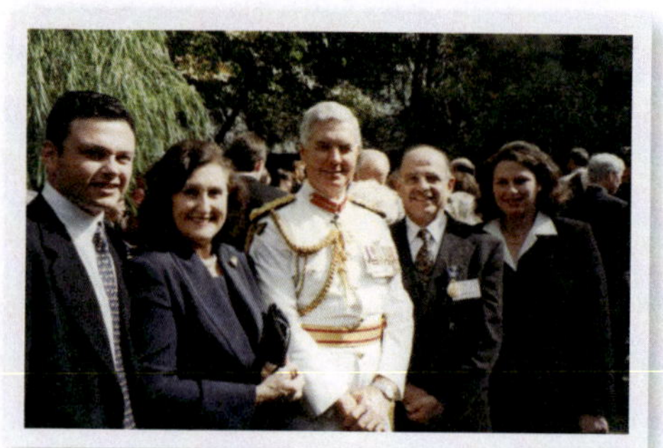

With Challis, Damon, Sasha and the Governor of Western Australia, Major General Philip Michael Jeffery.

Professor Ian Constable, head of the Lions Eye Institute, contacted me. Their chemist had developed an artificial cornea material, but the material needed to be transferred to a lens that could be transplanted onto the cornea. Constable needed someone to make his implants.

Because our laboratory had FDA approval, Professor Constable asked us to manufacture the artificial cornea for him. There is no other laboratory in the world that would have done this development work for him. We agreed to shape the material to create the artificial corneas, and they were successfully implanted. One day Constable called me and asked for all our lathing data and the procedures we had developed for manufacturing the artificial cornea. I declined!

Shortly after this I visited Pangolin, the company in Denver that supplied our lens blanks. It was owned by Bill Hoffman. Bill told me that a laboratory in Denver was making artificial corneas for the Lions Eye Institute. This was news to me! When I returned to Perth I called Professor Constable and told him what I had learned. He mumbled something to the effect that he was going to call me. I told him that we could not do any more work for him. At the time we were also making implants with the same material for patients with enunciated eyes, and Constable asked that we continue manufacturing them. I said we would not do anything further for him! The artificial cornea product was subsequently sold by Constable to CooperVision and nothing further was heard of the product.

CHAPTER ELEVEN

TRITON BIFOCAL LENS

The Translating Bifocal Lens

All soft bifocal lenses are of a simultaneous vision design that incorporate a central reading portion and a peripheral distance portion, or vice versa. These designs are generally described as a compromise for patient's vision.

I had designed a 'rigid translating bifocal' lens design we called the 'Linear Plus Bifocal' lens, made in a rigid gas permeable material that worked very well and provided patients with clear vision at all distances without compromise. I wanted to make a soft translating bifocal lens similar to the rigid lens. This was not easy with the DAC lathes and mill we had at the time. In May 2001 we bought a new lathe with an oscillating tool from DAC. This allowed us to make rigid gas permeable (RGP) translating bifocal lenses and toric lenses, and to develop the soft translating bifocal lens.

Triton

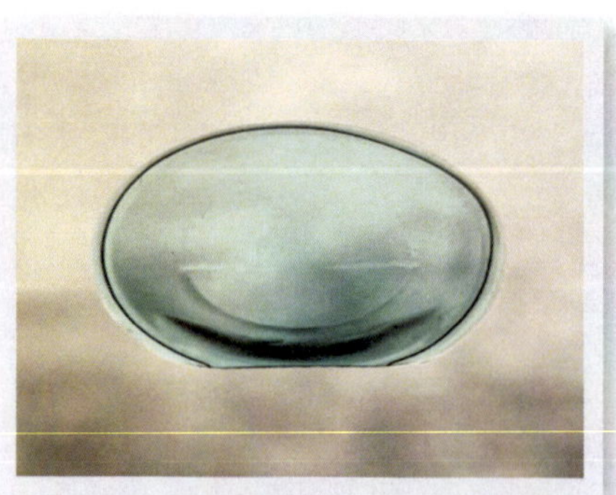

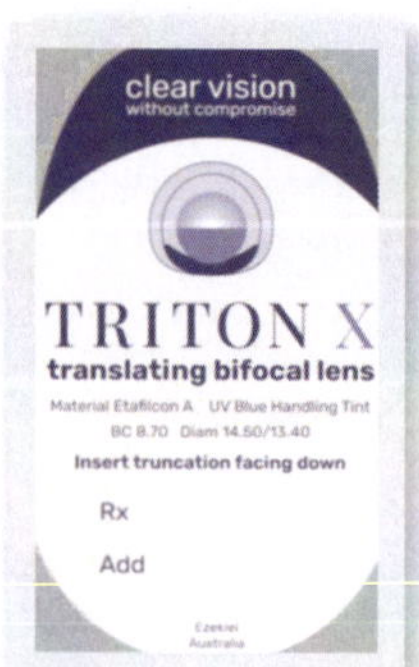

The soft translating bifocal lenses we made were translating well but the rounding of the junction of the truncation and ledge had to be done by hand (I mistakenly thought this would be done on the mill when it could have been done with the oscillating ALM lathe!). This caused reproducibility and comfort problems, but even so orders from the USA were growing. We applied to the FDA for approval for the translating bifocal lens and this was obtained 5th February 2003.

In June 2004 patents for the translating bifocal lens were received for Australia and the USA. Subsequently patents have been received for the manufacturing process in all major countries, and two for the USA. The European patent was applied for at the same time that I applied for patents in all other countries. It is not unknown for the patent process to take years – and it did! In early 2023, the patent examiner replied with objections to our application. He clearly didn't understand the reasons our application was so innovative – achieving a soft lens to translate, resulting in a soft translating bifocal lens. Together with a local patent attorney we sent a reply detailing why my application was unique. In June 2023 I was advised that my patent application had been approved in full.

Cast Moulding Laboratory

In 2003 I received an email from a gentleman in Korea, Wallis Kim. He said that another Korean, Andrew Kim, who had established three cast moulding laboratories, wanted to get out of Korea and come to Perth to set up a laboratory for us. We corresponded and Wallis and Andrew Kim visited us in Perth. We did our sums and Wallis told me he could sell all the lenses we made. (I never learn!). The market for contact lenses had moved to disposable lenses, and as I had always wanted to make these lenses, I took the opportunity. We nominated Andrew as a migrant and purchased the equipment to start a cast moulding line. The machines were standard Sumitomo moulding machines from Japan. Sailor Japan manufactured the machine that put the lens together, with robots that take the moulded parts, filled them with monomer and automatically placed them on a moving conveyor into a heating oven, to allow polymerisation to occur.

Designed by Andrew and purpose-built in Japan by Sailor, it took three months to make and deliver. In the meantime, we built a small clean room and moved the custom lenses for the final quality lens checking into this room. The old clean room was then used to accommodate the new cast moulding line.

I applied for a government grant to set up a cast moulding facility to cast mould the Triton bifocal lens. The custom bifocal lens worked well, but the market wanted disposable lenses. We were fortunate and received a government grant of $1.5 million, which we had to match over two years. It was a great help.

CHAPTER TWELVE

FAMILY continued

Paul and Tanya

Paul met Tanya Kiskanyan at Cornell. In 2000 they married at a golf course in Mt Tremblant, north of Montreal in Canada. Challis and I attended the wedding together with Sasha and her family, Damon and his wife Tania, the Eastwoods, the Silberts and the Steinbergs.

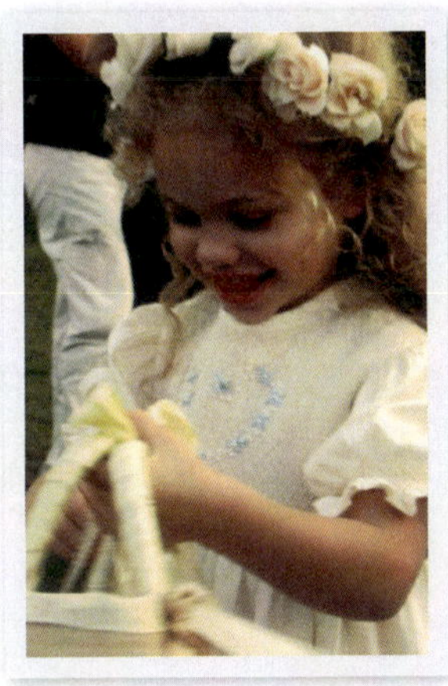

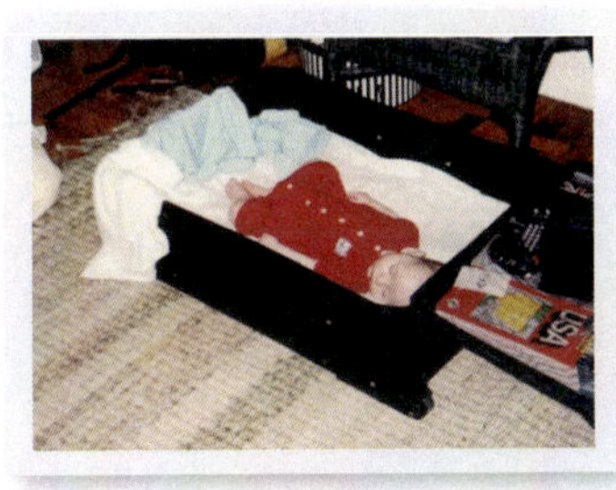

Olivia flower girl at Tanya and Paul's wedding.

Baby Max slept in a suitcase.

Paul and his friend Dave Rogers established a company in the renewable energy field based in Toronto called AMP. Paul works long hours and deserves to do well.

He has always been interested in music. He plays the piano and had DJ lessons in New York.

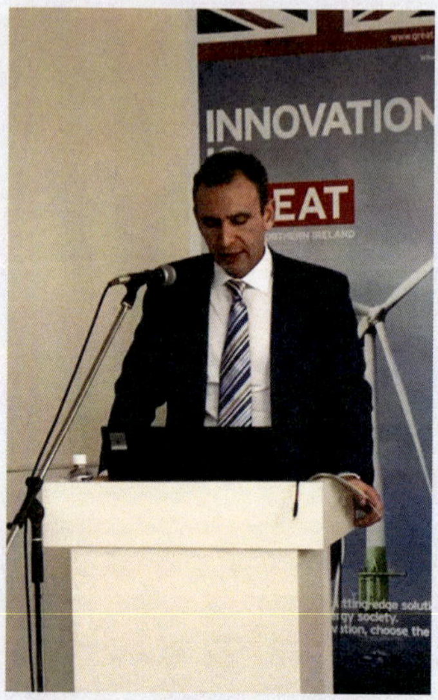

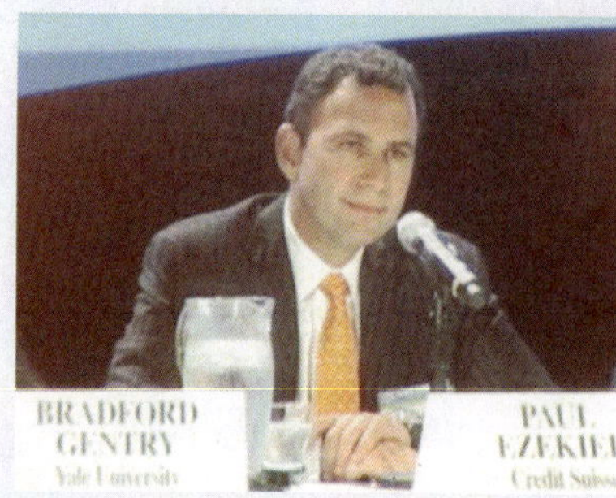

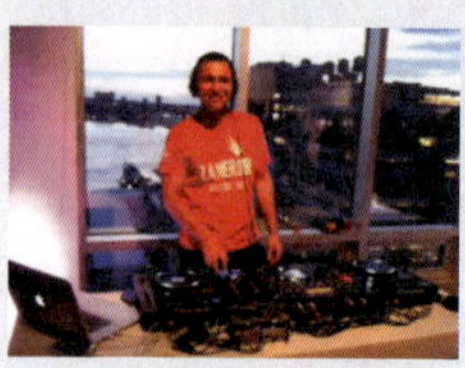

Paul establishing AMP, speaking at a conference and working as a DJ.

Birth of Olivia

Soon after Sasha and Russell married they flew to Ottawa, where Russell had a year on exchange. Sasha had a lovely girl named Olivia in May 2000. Challis, Paul, Tanya and I flew up from New York for the birth.

Pets

When we lived in Viking Road Dalkeith, we had a pet pink-and-grey parrot that Paul named Roy. He would fly around the family area, sit on our shoulders and nibble our ear lobes. Paul taught him to say a few words. One day we were at a pet store and saw a chain that could fasten to a bird's leg, and onto the ground, allowing it to feed on the lawn but not fly away. Perfect for Roy. Unfortunately the first time we tried it Roy took off, never to be seen again.

We loved our dogs. All were standard or miniature poodles. We bred Irma, one of our standard poodles. The night she was to deliver, Robin, our dog groomer, came to help. She placed a towel on the warm electric fry pan and placed the twelve pups on the towel as they were born. Sadly, one died at birth. In the morning Paul came to tell us another one had died but not to worry as he had put the dead pup in the fry pan and it was turned to hot!

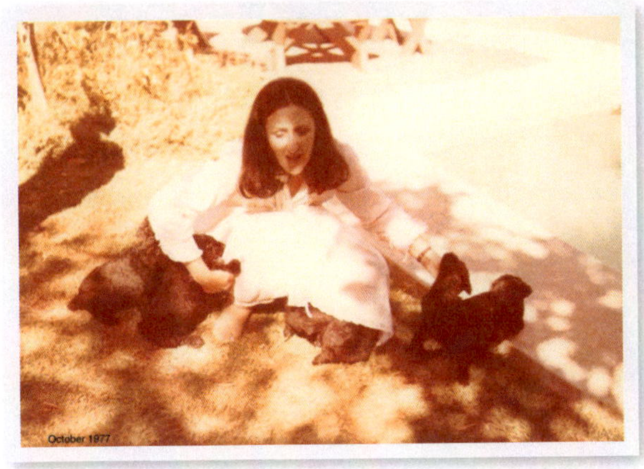

With Elle and her litter.

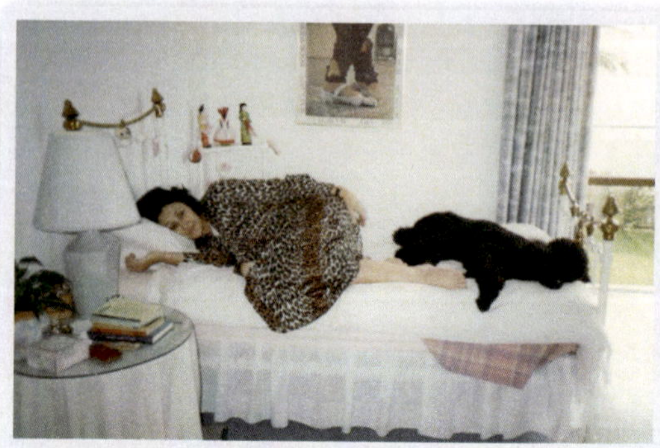

Challis with Elle.

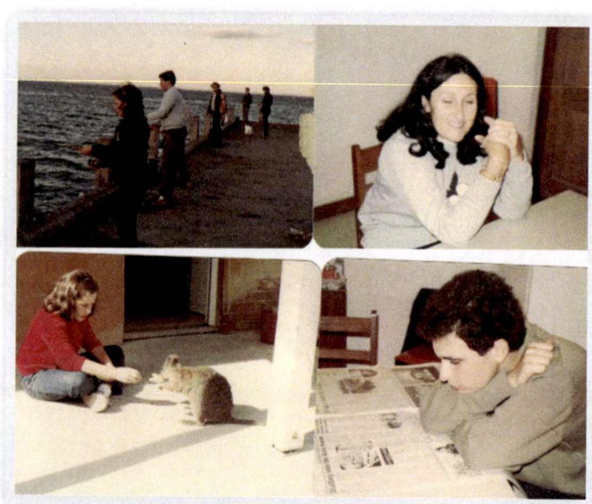

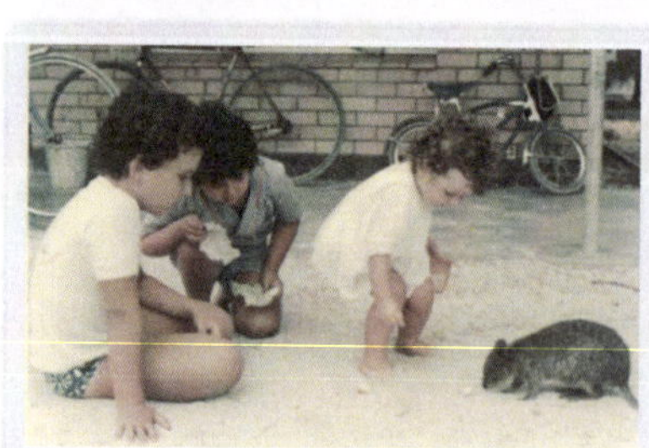

Family holidays on Rottnest Island.

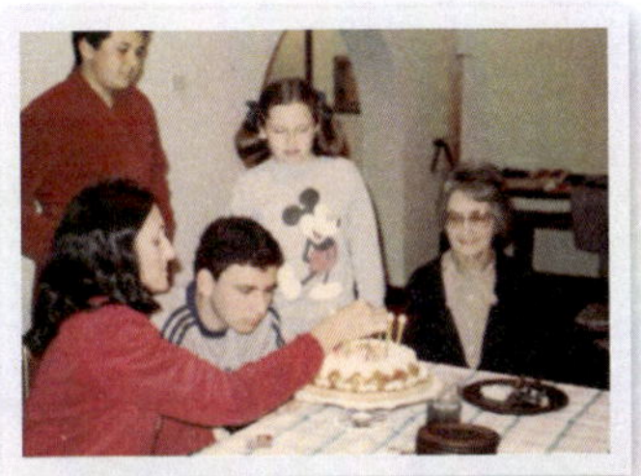

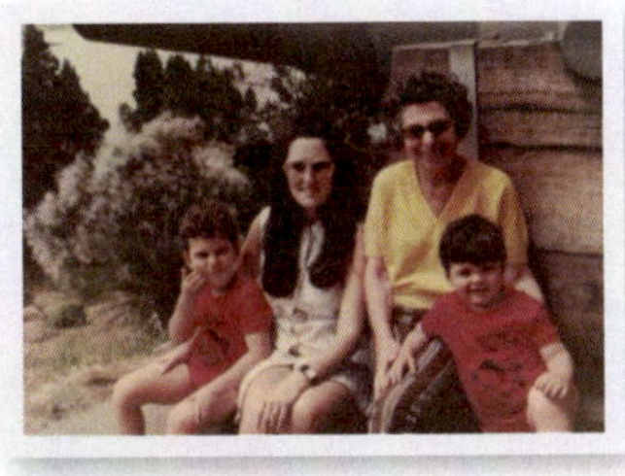

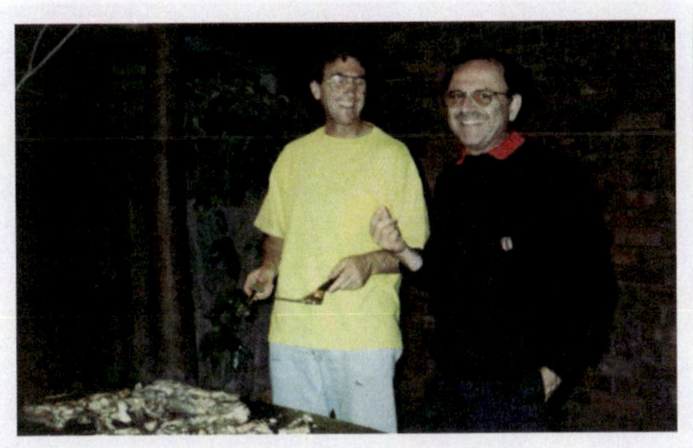

Challis with her mother Nan Connell, 1982.

Challis with my mother, 1969.

With Barry Silbert in Yallingup, 1991.

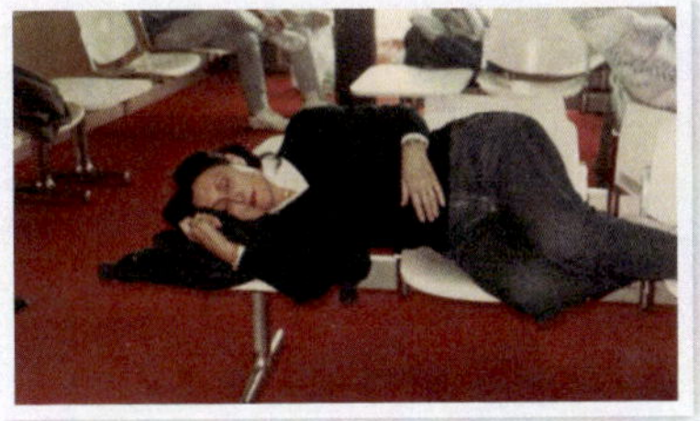

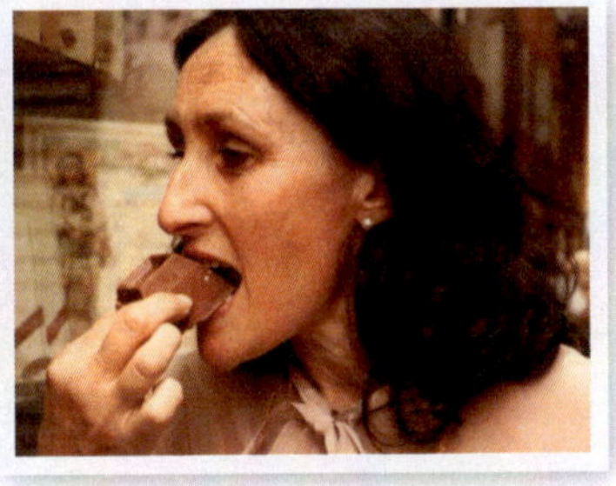

Challis's travels.

Leeuwin Concerts

The Leeuwin Estate winery in Margaret River held annual concerts with prominent overseas artists. We enjoyed the outings, and would get there early to get a good spot near the stage on the lawn with friends, where we had a picnic dinner with wine. In 1992 Diana Ross performed. This is a review of the concert, mentioning Paul.

Diana such a spec-tacle

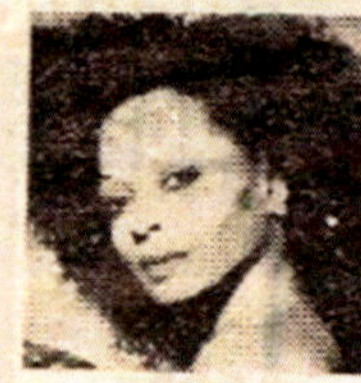

☐ Diana Ross

DIANA Ross needs glasses! That's what Perth optometrist Damon Ezekiel was thinking to himself at the Leeuwin Estate concert last week.

During one of her walks into the Leeuwin crowd, Miss Ross headed towards the Ezekiel party which included Damon's brother, Dr Paul Ezekiel.

Much to the chagrin of Damon, the former Supreme ignored him and singled out Dr Ezekiel.

Dr Ezekiel stood up and walked towards Miss Ross who gave the normally reserved doctor a big kiss and a hug.

Dr Ezekiel's mother and father Chalice and Don, who were also at the concert, were equally surprised by the actions of their normally shy but laconic son.

While in his clinch with Miss Ross, Dr Ezekiel was heard to exclaim: "Oh Diana"... sounds like a cue for another song!

Fishing

I love fishing. In 1999 I went fishing in Canada with a group from Perth that included my good friend Malcolm Steinberg. We flew to Vancouver, then flew another hour north and then by helicopter to the Langara Fishing Lodge. It was a lovely experience and I actually caught some fish! Our group each put in $100 and the person who caught the most fish received the prize. Unbelievably I won!

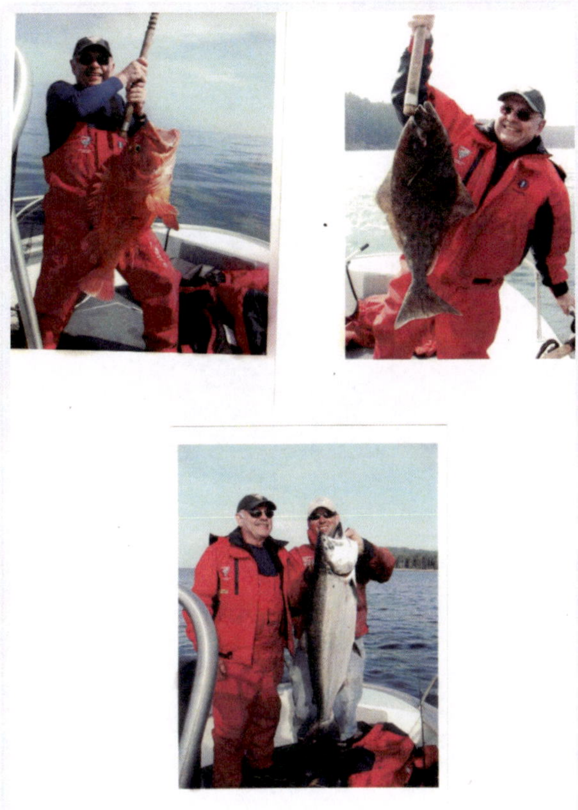

With some of the fish I caught.

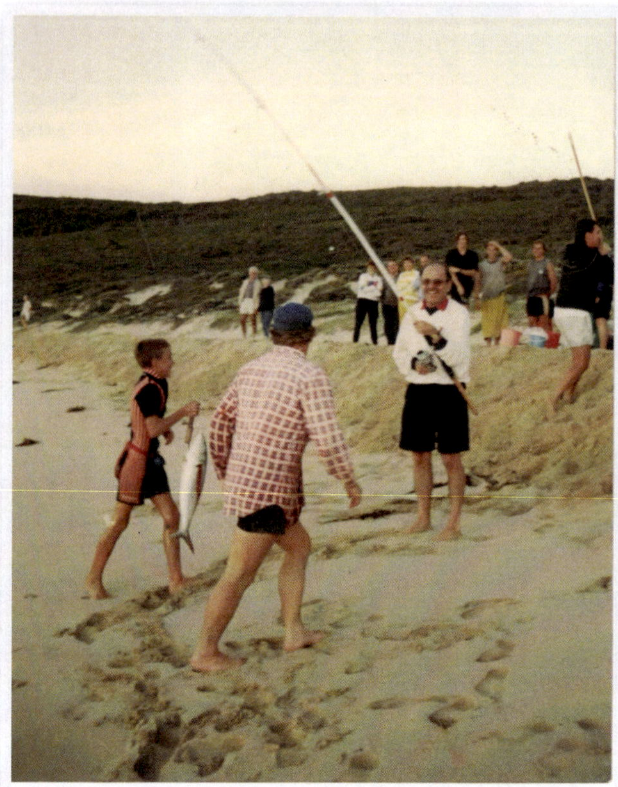

Fishing at Yallingup.

My 70th birthday.

Paul surprised me and arrived unexpectedly for my 70th birthday, in September 2006. Sasha organised a surprise dinner for all the family at the Kailas fish restaurant in North Perth.

CHAPTER THIRTEEN
PROFESSIONAL CHALLENGES

David Masel

I was concerned that the new cast moulding plant was going to be costlier than I expected, so I called Michael Cohen, an old friend who had several companies, to ask how I could raise money. He suggested that maybe I needed someone to help with managing the laboratory. It was 2005, and I was then 69 years of age. The succession plan I had hoped for with Damon was not going to materialise, so I responded that this would be well worth looking at. Michael's brother-in-law, David Masel, had just left from a management position and was looking at other options. He was only interested to join if he could have equity. We met, together with Paul. Masel seemed a good person so we agreed. He would get equity in the lab. He would put in only $200,000, but our investment was in the person, not the cash. He has turned out to be an excellent hard worker. It was such a relief for me to have someone I felt I could trust with the laboratory as a priority. Little did I know that he would later engineer a group to buy the laboratory, to my detriment. So it apparently does not pay to be too trusting!

Manufacturing Soft Lens Materials

We were buying our RGP and soft blanks from a small lab in Denver called Pangolin, owned and run by Bill and Renata Hoffman. Bill had previously made RGP materials, but was caught up in a patent problem and barred for some years to making RGP materials. When the restriction was over he started to make lens materials again. We must have been one of his earliest accounts. I visited Bill one day in Denver and during our meeting he asked me why I wasn't making my own soft lens materials. I told him that it was too difficult. He ran me through the process and told me it wasn't. I asked him how much it would cost for him to teach me, and he said just a ticket for him and his wife Renata to visit Perth sometime. So we sent a technician over to Denver and he was taught the process on how to make soft lens materials. Bill told us where to source the raw materials and even gave us some blue dye to add a handling tint in lenses that J&J gave him to use on a project. And Bill was selling us soft lens blanks! Really very good of him. We became self-sufficient in making our own soft lens materials and must have been one of the only contact lens laboratories to do so.

Bill and Renata visited us here in Perth and thoroughly enjoyed themselves.

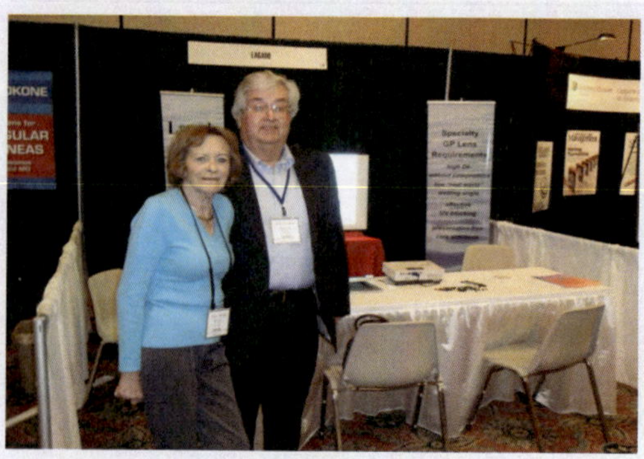

Bill and Renata Hoffman.

Scleral Lenses

In 1984, The American Academy of Optometry invited me to speak on scleral lenses:

F.A. A.O.

AMERICAN ACADEMY of OPTOMETRY

THE CORNEA AND CONTACT LENS SECTION

CHAIRMAN
MICHAEL G. HARRIS, O.D., M.S.
School of Optometry
University of California
Berkeley, California 94720
415-642-5781

SECTION EXECUTIVE COMMITTEE

IMMEDIATE PAST PRESIDENT
SHELDON WECHSLER, M. Opt., O.D.

VICE CHAIRMAN
RICHARD D. BRANNEN, O.D.

SECRETARY
C.A. BAYSHORE, O.D.

PROGRAM CHAIRMAN
RODGER T. KAME, O.D.

COURSES CHAIRMAN

DIPLOMATE AWARD CHAIRMAN
GERALD E. LOWTHER, O.D., Ph.D.

CASE REPORTS CHAIRMAN
STEPHEN LEXXER, O.D.

March 15, 1984

Donald Ezekiel, O.D.
Western Australia Contact Lens Manufacturing
43 Outram Street
West Perth, Australia 6005

Dear Doctor Ezekiel:

As a result of a recent conversation with Dr. Melvin Remba, I write to ask if you might be interested in reporting on your experience on the application and efficacy of gas permeable scleral lenses. The contact lens program of the American Academy of Optometry is to be held on Tuesday morning December 11, 1984 in St. Louis, Missouri. The symposium is entitled "Contemporary and Innovative Contact Lens Procedures".

Even though the concept of the gas permeable sclerals have been discussed in the past, I understand you have taken the initiative and implemented this concept.

The Cornea and Contact Lens Section would be honored to have you present a lecture of approximately one-half hour as part of this symposium.

I look forward to hearing from you. A reply by April 15, would be greatly appreciated.

Sincerely,

Rodger T. Kame, O.D., F.A.A.O.
Program Chairman
RTK/ii

SECTION COMMITTEE

MICHAEL FRIEDBERG, O.D.
MORTON KAY, O.D.
DONALD KORB, O.D.
CLARENCE L. McEACHERN, O.D.
DONALD A. SPRINGER, O.D.
CHARLES STEWART, O.D., Ph.D.
SOL TABAK, O.D.
C. EDWARD WILLIAMS, O.D.

AND ALL PAST CHAIRMEN

Gas Permeable Scleral Lens

Mary Bremner, the senior ophthalmologist at Princess Margaret Hospital for Children, was trained in the UK and knew the benefits of scleral lenses. She would call almost weekly to tell me that she had just removed a cataract from a baby's eye and would I come to the hospital in two days' time and fit a scleral lens. I would go to the hospital, gown up and take a mould of the anaesthetised baby's eye. When the eye closes, Bell's Phenomenon occurs, where the eye rolls up under the top lid. I would invariably take a mould of the lower fornix of the eye with little impression of the cornea. There had to be a better way!

Rigid corneal lenses were no longer being manufactured in a non-pervious PMMA material, but in new breathing gas permeable (GP) materials. Why were we using PMMA material and not the GP materials for our scleral lens patients? Maybe it would make life easier for paediatric patients, their parents and for me, as the GP material could help in getting a faster and better result.

Polymer Technology in Boston was our source of GP materials. I flew to Boston and sat with the then owners of Polymer Technology, Perry Rosenthal and Lou Major, and asked them for large blanks. Perry asked why I wanted large blanks, and I told him I was making scleral lenses. Perry, who was head ophthalmologist of the contact lens clinic at the Massachusetts Eye and Ear Hospital, responded that "no-one fits scleral lenses anymore!" I told him that this was not so, and that there was a need for this material to be used for scleral lenses.

Lou Major was responsible for the laboratory and he eventually said he would make large blanks for me. Nothing eventuated! The promised large blanks did not arrive. I would telex Lou two or three times a week asking for the blanks. He later told me he had an ever-growing pile of telexes on his desk. He made a rod in a large diameter GP material and sent it to me, and we cut it into blanks and made scleral lenses. I refitted happy PMMA scleral lens patients with the scleral lenses made from the GP material. All patients reported the lenses to be more comfortable than the PMMA lenses they were wearing.

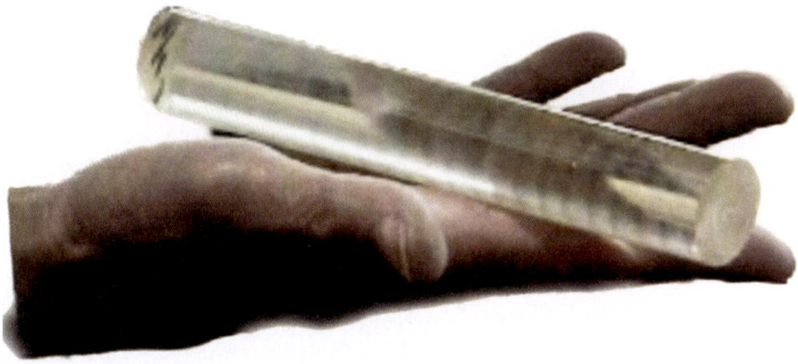

The first large diameter gas permeable material suitable for manufacturing in a scleral lens was supplied in a rod form. Today, materials used for scleral lens manufacture are sold as small buttons, with just enough material to lathe a single scleral lens.

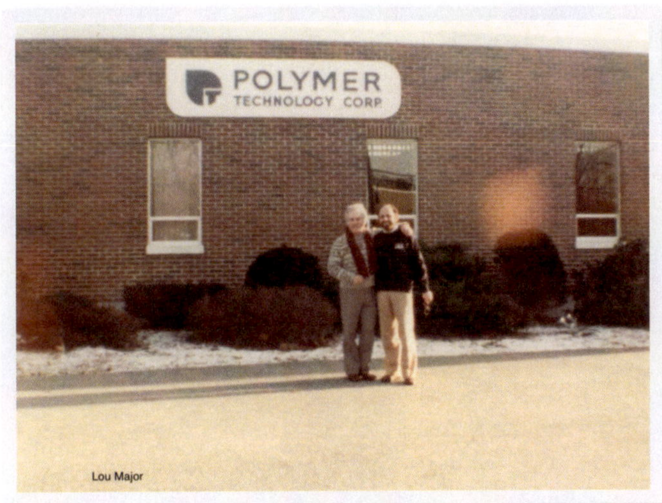

With Lou Major at Polymer Technology.

My family had accompanied me on the trip to Boston, and while we were there, Lou and his wife Beverly took Challis and I and the children skiing to Vermont. They collected clothing for the cold and for skiing and Lou taught us how to ski. The children took to it - Challis and I were not so good. On one occasion we took the ski lift and when we got off the lift, we landed badly and collapsed into a pile onto the ground, much to the hilarity of the children following in the next chair. The lift was stopped while we scrambled out of the way. Somehow we managed to get down. End of our skiing! A safer time was spent having a coffee in the restaurant.

The first paper on the use of gas permeable material for scleral lenses was presented in 1963, at the annual meeting of the British Contact Lens Society. It was titled, 'Gas Permeable Materials to Manufacture Haptic Lenses'. The link to the full paper can be read in the Appendix.

The conclusion stated:

> The Boston gas permeable haptic lens is an advance for the haptic lens practitioner and his patient. For the practitioner, the lens is very much easier and quicker to fit. For the patient, the lens appears to be a more comfortable and acceptable lens than the PMMA haptic lens. These factors suggest that the haptic lens will once again be more readily available for those patients for whom it still remains the lens of choice.

Irving Fatt was the world authority on oxygen permeability. He presented at an ISCLS congress, and later reported on the meeting, writing in the magazine *Optician*, "many in the audience did not believe that the GP material would make any difference to oxygen transmission to the eye owing to the thickness needed to manufacture the lens."

I subsequently read a paper at a meeting of the ISCLS in France. I showed a video I made on the GP lens fitting process that included patients with a range of ocular conditions where a scleral lens was their only option to obtain clear and comfortable vision. Irving Fatt was at the meeting. After my paper he told me that I was clearly getting results and if I would send him lenses and the lens design details, he would do some calculations on the oxygen permeability of the lens.

Irving reported that the eye received five times the oxygen than the eye needed. All correspondence from Irving is now at The Contact Lens Museum in Portland, USA.

My paper was subsequently published in the *Journal of the BCLA*. Perry read the paper and called me, asking if he could visit and would I show him what I was doing. Of course! Very few patients worldwide had the option of this wonderful lens. That someone of Perry's stature was interested in providing patients with this option was a huge plus.

I could have patented the idea, but there were so few practitioners offering the scleral lens. I was seeing in practice that the lens was very much needed and life-changing for patients, and was happy that the scleral option might be available for patients who had no other option to obtain vision and comfort.

Perry visited me in Perth and I showed him a range of patients who were wearing the GP scleral lens. We then went to the laboratory and I showed him how the lens was made and how lens modifications were done. No secrets, I was just happy that the scleral lens might be made more available to patients. Soon after he returned to Boston he messaged me asking where he could source the chucks needed to mount the large scleral lens. We had a metal lathe and a technician who made them for us, so we made a range of chucks and sent them to Perry, complimentary. He went on to establish the Boston Foundation, where scleral lens designs were developed. Perry introduced GP scleral lenses to the USA.

The GP scleral lens has invigorated and changed the rigid contact lens market and is now fitted worldwide. I spoke at a meeting on scleral lenses in 2019. The largest rigid lens US laboratory told me that 75% of all rigid lenses they made were now scleral lenses and this was growing.

I have been referred to as the 'Grandfather of the Gas Permeable Scleral Lens' and have since received several awards for my pioneering work. It was not clever, but an obvious progression for scleral lenses.

I have done several podcasts where I was asked what I would like to be remembered for. I replied that, "Our sages said we must leave the world in a better place than we found it, and I have tried." One interviewer, who was not Jewish, responded, "Wow!" That was great.

As practitioners worldwide started to contact me about how the lenses were fitted, I made, with professional help, a video showing the full fitting process. It showed patients with a series of ocular conditions wearing GP scleral lenses that without which, they would not have such vision and comfort.

The video concluded with the following statement:

> The advent of using gas permeable materials for the manufacture of scleral lenses has resulted in a scleral lens that was easier for the practitioner to fit and more comfortable for the patient to wear. These factors suggest that the gas permeable scleral lens will become more readily available for patients, for whom it remains the lens of choice to obtain vision.

Other Projects

I regularly had approaches from people who had ideas on lenses or materials. I always agreed to work with them - but they invariably did not work out, and came with a cost to us! But I felt we always learned something from the exercise.

A senior scientist at Dow Corning, Ned Gvozdic, made contact with Paul in 2004. He had ideas to make a silicon-hydrogel material with the properties that would overcome the problems the current S-H properties materials had. It could be patented, as the approach is very different to materials now available. We came to an agreement with him and financed him to do the work. In 2007 he filed for a patent.

Joe Barr is a prominent optometrist I have known for many years. He was previously the editor of *Contact Lens Spectrum,* a journal that I have contributed to, and he also did a workshop on scleral lenses when he was head at Ohio State University. Joe had been appointed to head Bausch & Lomb's R&D in contact lenses. I saw him at a meeting in Las Vegas in January 2008, and spoke to him about the materials project, for which we had applied for a patent. I asked if B&L would like to work with us on this project. He was very interested and in July, three B&L people, along with Paul, Ned and Bob McKeller (our patent guy) met in New York. They were interested and I felt it would be just wonderful if we worked together on the project.

In September 2008, they emailed to advise that they were not interested in pursuing the project. We would just have to keep looking, but with the worldwide economic downturn it wouldn't be easy. I spoke to prominent US optometrist Art Epstein. He suggested

Alcon might be interested, as he had a good relationship with them. He seemed to know what was going on with the other large labs and thought they would be good to work with. We communicated non-disclosure agreements but heard nothing further.

In early 2007 I had a call from Tan Le, founder and CEO of Emotiv, a bioinformatics and technology company, asking if we could make a part for a device out of polymer. He came to Perth and explained that they had developed a device that sits on a person's head and reads electrical impulses of thought, allowing the mind's intentions to be displayed on a screen. As I enjoy the challenges of research we made many devices in different hydrogel materials for him. Unfortunately, polymer materials lose their water content when exposed to air. With input from Ned we developed a material that retains its moisture for months. They forecast that in three years, they would need 400 million units a year. We applied for a patent on the material. We made many versions and the feedback is that it has remained moist after three months. The device was shown at trade shows, on the internet and television, and looked promising. We later learned that they had financial problems and had put off most of their staff. The project did not proceed further.

But then in November 2012 came this report from *Good News Israel*:

> Israeli biotechnology company X-trodes announced on Monday its partnership with San Francisco-based bioinformatics firm Emotiv to launch a first-of-its-kind medical-grade wearable solution for brain and physiological monitoring outside of clinical settings. Emotiv customers can now use X-trodes' proprietary dry-printed electrodes to stream user-generated data through the EmotivPRO mobile app for processing and analysis on Emotiv's cloud-based platform.

So it looked like Emotiv was still alive and doing well. Another case of 'if only'?

Chiron Laboratory, based in Irving, California, asked us to make small diameter lenses for cornea implanting to create a reading portion after IOL implantation. Clinical trials were done in Brazil by ophthalmologist Richard Keates, who incidentally was the specialist who visited us in Perth to evaluate the IOGEL lens for Alcon. Early results were promising. I visited Chiron in Irving to be updated on the project.

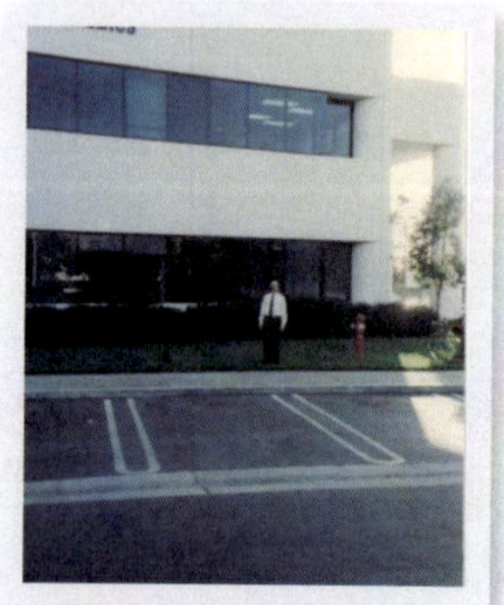

Outside Chiron Laboratory.

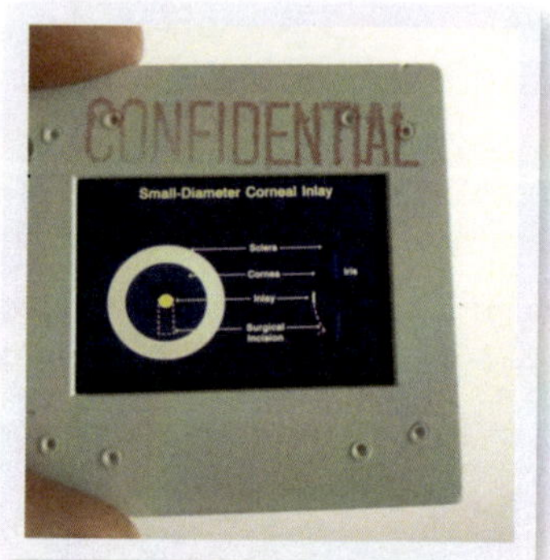

The small diameter corneal lens.

In April 2009, we had an email from a group in the USA who connected people in industries that could help each other. They had a client who was looking to see if there was any R&D on a material that didn't lose water. Ned's material fit the description. We sent them details and they wanted to discuss the project further. Was it J&J?

It was. In our discussions with them we mentioned the bifocal lens we had developed. They were interested, but they are a huge company. It wouldn't be easy getting through their systems.

Contact lens for Cattle

I received a call from a vet at Curtin University who had a project trying to treat cattle getting red eye from abrasions while they fed from wheat stalks. A few drops of antibiotics clear the infection up. He thought that a contact lens soaked in an antibiotic worn by the cattle would be a good fix.

We made large bandage lenses in a high water content material that we used for extended wear, and tinted them so we could check if the lenses were still in place in the cattle's eyes.

Cattle have a nictitating (third) membrane that moves when blinking so the insertion of the lens was tricky. I went to the university where the vet had a cow in a pen. He put his fingers up its nostrils and the cow became paralysed. The lens insertion went well and then the vet said he would try it, and would I do the necessary holding of the cow's nostril. I replied sorry, but no!

Unfortunately the drug was not bound to the lens and was lost from the lens after just a day. The project aborted.

Financial Problems

By 2009 the world's economic problems had come to Australia. St George Bank, who were very good in helping us establish the cast moulding laboratory, advised us that they now were not interested in continuing to support us. Although they had more than enough security with our property guarantees, they wouldn't lend us any more money and in fact did not want us as an account. In addition, the licence to sell lenses in China was taking a long time, and we needed it before we could legally sell in China. In the meantime, J&J and Ciba were evaluating the Triton lens.

This all caused us great stress. Accounts were not being paid and we were stretching our creditors as long as possible. It became such a problem that we were looking to sell part of the lab to possible equity partners. Finding anyone interested in Perth would be a problem. Money was scarce.

We decided to sell our Yallingup beach house. Challis loves the beach, but because of her health problems the house was rarely used. We had built the beach house and enjoyed many years and happy times there. It was next door to Barry and Bev Silbert's house, which was nice as they are good friends. But with finances tight, Yallingup had to be sold. The sale would provide the cash so the lab could survive by marketing our products.

By 2010, the bifocal lens was getting attention, but it would be some time before we would get any benefit from a licence agreement. In the meantime we were struggling to pay bills to get product out the door. Because the St George Bank would no longer assist us, we had to sell the Hutton Street property, where the laboratory was located, to clear borrowings. The sale would clear debts and make the attraction of equity easier. It was a very stressful time for Challis and me.

In April 2011 we sold the Hutton Street premises to the Mazda dealer next door. I had offered it to him for more than the going price, as I knew he wanted the property to expand his business.

Becoming Vertically Integrated

In the manufacturing process of soft lens materials, an initiator is needed for polymerisation to occur. We initially managed to get this in a powder form from the Lions Eye Institute when we made our lathed soft lens materials. But in the cast moulding process the initiator has to be in a liquid form, which is very volatile and extremely expensive to ship by air due to its explosive properties. It requires a special handling container. To ship a small quantity from Korea cost US$18,000 for each container, and this would last just six weeks. Through Andrew Kim's network he found a source in Korea where, for a fee, he would teach us the process to manufacture the initiator. Andrew Kim and Darren Walker - the technician who was making our polymers after spending time with Bill Hoffman - went to South Korea and learned the process of making the initiator. We purchased the necessary equipment and began making the initiator in-house. The result was excellent and a big saving.

So now we were self-sufficient, being vertically integrated in making both lens materials for custom lenses and for the cast moulding lenses.

The Batam Laboratory, Indonesia

When we started cast moulding lenses we realised that Wallis Kim had only told us about the front end of the manufacturing process, which made the lens but was still in its shell. A further process was needed to open the shell and extract the lens, check the lens quality and then package the lens. We started to do this in Perth, but soon realised that it was very labour intensive and with our high wage system in Australia would not be viable.

Wallis Kim suggested we do it in Batam, Indonesia, a 45-minute ferry ride from Singapore, as staff was cheaper than in Australia. Masel went to Batam with Wallis and rented a small factory space there. In ten days it was fitted out with a tiled floor, partitioned and air conditioned. We soon realised that it was far too small. Another costly Masel contribution.

A laboratory in Batam that did lens checking and packaging had closed and been empty for nine months. The owners had spent $300,000 setting it up, so we rented the property and purchased all the equipment, over a period of time, for $280,0000. Masel negotiated the price down by just $20,000! My fault. I should have been involved.

An automatic lens packaging machine was ordered from an Australian supplier and shipped to Batam, so that all the back-end processes could be undertaken there. The materials we were using for standard lenses in a polymer had been superseded by new silicon-hydrogel materials, so the lenses we made were not easy to sell. Coloured contact lenses were quite popular, and as they attracted a premium, we started to make the coloured lens in the hydrogel material. The colour printing is a manual process, but staff was cheap in Indonesia.

Masel found a local marketing group who he said did the Singapore Air marketing (?). They put together a marketing package on the lenses. Again, this Masel decision was costly as the work they did was awful and a total waste of money. Future displays and marketing were better.

The Sale of Gelflex

None of our efforts to sell the lab were successful. David Masel spoke to a friend, David Swartz, who made an offer. When the bank wanted out from our account, Masel made out that a sale was urgent. We came to an arrangement with Swartz, and he acquired the laboratory for just $360,000. It wasn't a good deal for us and it cost us a lot, but it was an out for me. When I told Masel I had been screwed, he replied that, "at least you will be famous." I told him that wouldn't provide food on the table.

Going through my files sometime later, I came across some papers and found out that Masel had tried to get a group in China interested in the lab. His pitch for a 50% share included a valuation of the lab for $US2.5 million!

The cost of establishing the cast moulding facility was over $3 million. We had help with a government grant to pay half of this, *plus* all the manufacturing and inspection gear, *plus* trained staff and goodwill ... none of which was taken into account.

All I retained were the patents for the bifocal lens and my antique optical collection. Masel would end up with 25% of the laboratory and Graham Barrett 12.5%. The legal agreement that Swartz sent to me left out one paragraph that was in our favour and added several that chipped away and wanted guarantees for four years against anything and everything. Fortunately, I had an excellent lawyer in Andrew Throssell, who was very thorough. I spent several hours with him going through the agreement and he rewrote it.

When the lab was sold, there was an outstanding problem with the quality of the lenses sent to China. They had rightly rejected lenses that never should have been sent. They were to be returned for a credit of $45,694.54. Once the lenses had been returned and checked, then the $45,694.54 would be deducted from the monies owed to me. Masel told me that he didn't trust the Chinese as the lenses returned may include lenses we did not supply.

When Masel advised the lenses had been returned to Batam I told him that I, together with my accountant, wanted to audit them.

Masel told me he would arrange accommodation and transport from the Batam wharf. We flew to Singapore and caught the ferry to Batam, where the local Gelflex manager Pascal Segar picked us up and asked why we were there. Apparently, all the boxes with the vials containing the lenses had been opened and put together into jars. Coloured lenses are different with each design having different prices. There was no way we could do an audit with jars full of mixed lenses.

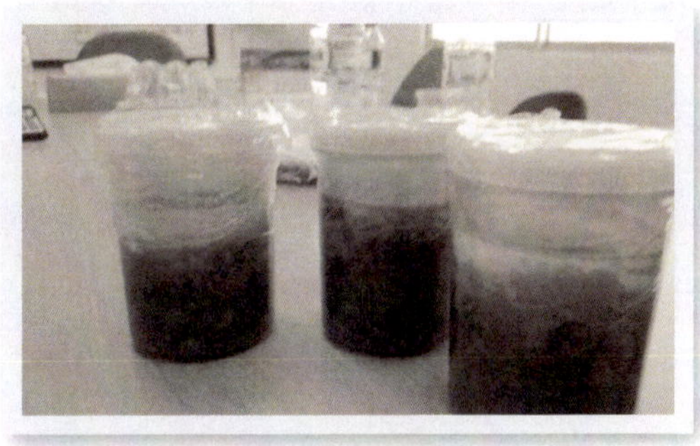

Lenses all mixed up in jars.

On my return I sent Masel a letter detailing the waste of time and money this trip had been, and included an invoice for our costs. There was nothing to audit - which he would have been aware of. He brushed it aside and told me I should have trusted him! Showed what type of a person he was!

Masel continued to pump me for information on custom lenses. On many occasions during the five years he was at the lab, he had said the custom lab should be shut down. He spent nothing on it, but came to realise that it could make money only if an effort was put in.

Several years after the laboratory was sold I ran into Graham Barratt, who had become a shareholder in the lab. I asked him how the lab was going. "Not too well," he replied, "they have products that other labs have." I told him the reason the cast moulding lab was established was to make the bifocal lens, and the market for the lens was substantial. He asked would I be interested to talk to them. I replied NO! I didn't trust them.

The settlement of the lab acquisition occurred on 20th June 2010. I was kept on as a consultant for four hours a day with a cap of

$10,000 a month for twelve months. The interaction with Masel was on a need-to-know basis, with no contact at all with Swartz. I enjoyed the shorter working day. It meant I could have an afternoon sleep and get my affairs in order.

When we won the Small Business Award I had been approached by several businesspeople who were interested in investing in the laboratories. Perhaps I should have looked for a good investor; it may well have had a very different outcome.

CHAPTER FOURTEEN
OVERSEAS TRAVEL

Cruising to Israel

After the lab was sold I booked a holiday to the US and then a Mediterranean cruise on a 6-star ship, the *Silverseas,* that would call into Israeli ports. It would be nice to see the family again.

Three weeks before we were due to leave, Challis developed a very bad lung infection. I called the head microbiologist at Sir Charles Gardiner hospital, Clay Golledge, and he took a sputum sample to his lab. He called us on the Sunday night. Challis had a bad fungal lung infection. He put her on medication, and fortunately it worked. Over the years Clay has been a wonderful and caring doctor in his continuing care for Challis.

We first flew to New York. Paul managed to find a very good pulmonary physiotherapist for Challis and this made a huge difference to her health. We then flew to Frankfurt and onto Athens, where we stayed overnight. The hotel we had booked and paid for in Athens was overbooked and after some time we were directed to another hotel. This is Greece! Next day we caught a taxi to Piraeus and boarded the ship for the cruise. The cruise on the *Silverseas* was wonderful and did us both the world of good. The ship called into a port almost every day, but we didn't go on any side trips. We usually went ashore and walked to towns, enjoyed a coffee and looked at the shops. In Kusadasi, a Turkish port, we called at a shop selling 'Genuine Copy Watches.' We bought a copy watch for Sasha and a silk carpet for us. The ship then stopped at Ashkelon in Israel, and left next day from Haifa. We got off the ship in Ashkelon and caught a taxi to Rivka's home in Tel Aviv where we spent the night.

Rivka and all the children took us out for dinner to a seaside restaurant. It was lovely and great to be with family. The next day Ron and Guy took the day off from work to take me to Jerusalem. Rivka told them not to go to the Muslim quarter of the old city as there was a disturbance the previous day. We went straight to the

Muslim quarter and spent three-and-a-half hours walking the old city, having lunch in an orthodox market. It was marvellous. In the evening we went to Guy's home where all the family had gathered for dinner, and from there we caught a taxi to Haifa and reboarded the ship. We must spend more time in Israel and with the family. They are a lovely family and made us very welcome.

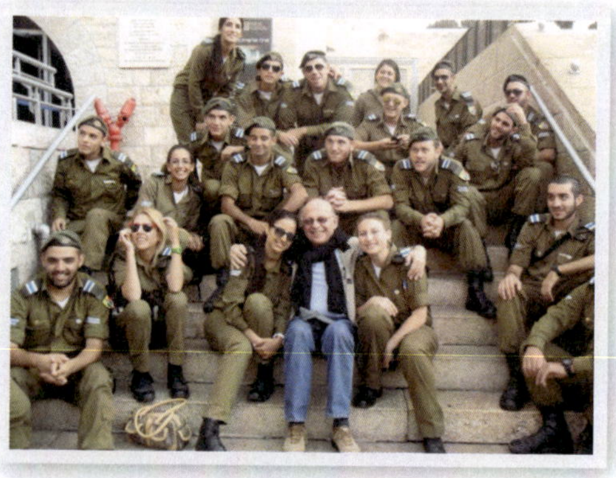

At the entrance to the Wailing Wall.

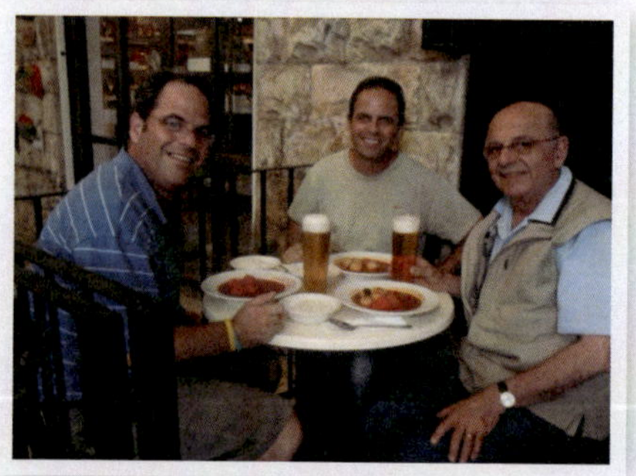

With nephews Ron and Guy in Jerusalem.

Schmuel Berman

While in Tel Aviv I visited Schmuel Berman. Schmuel was an optometrist who made his own contact lenses. He had visited us in Perth several years earlier to learn what I was doing with scleral lenses, and we corresponded frequently and exchanged ideas. He had been unwell with blood cancer and was on a research drug designed to prevent it progressing. He was a very good and innovative optometrist with a lovely practice and a small lens laboratory within the practice. We had lunch together. It was good to see him again.

Later that year he passed away. He was such a good person. Very sad. He will be missed.

We got off the ship in Istanbul. Our travel agent, Valerie Berman, is the daughter of Margaret Proud, my lovely old secretary. When she did our booking she told me that one night in Istanbul was not long enough, so we stayed for three days. We should have stayed longer. It was great and we would love to go back.

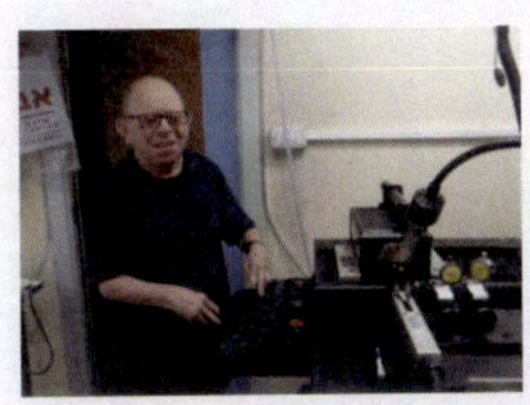

Schmuel at his practice and laboratory.

Before we had left home, once our US travel dates had been finalised, I had emailed the big four cast moulding laboratories in the USA. I told them what I had developed with the bifocal lens and said if they were interested, I would visit and make a presentation and demonstration of the lens. Three laboratories replied by return email, saying they looked forward to my visit. The fourth, Cooper Vision, were not interested, telling me I wouldn't be welcome as I am a competitor manufacturer. "No problem," I told them - but I'm not sure who I was competing against!

So in January 2013 I landed in New York and visited the major laboratories who were interested in the bifocal lens.

Pitching the Bifocal Lens in the US

The first laboratory I visited was Johnson and Johnson in Jacksonville. I arrived early at eleven am; the meeting was scheduled for two pm. I was met at reception and asked if I would like to go back to the hotel and someone would pick me up for the meeting. While I was waiting to go the hotel a Pat Adams came and said he would take me to lunch. He was a very nice guy. I thought he was just someone from their group and later found that he is head Director of Product Development at J&J. Over lunch I told him that the lab was sold and that I didn't do well out of it, but had retained the patents. He told me he thought I had done really well from the deal. I hoped he was right!

After lunch we returned to the facility. There were three people present: Pat Adams; Kurt Moody, Senior Optometrist and Director, Design Platform Research; and Geoffrey Roffman, Patent Director. I did my presentation but not a demonstration. They were very interested and positive and said they would get back to me. Within a week Pat emailed me a term sheet. What I really liked about them is that they were positive about what I had. In the term sheet they spelled out what they would do in year one, year two and so on.

Over many months I had several further emails and discussions with J&J. Pat Adams was moved aside and dealmaker Ed Rastrelli was now taking over negotiations. One email told me that they couldn't justify the money to move ahead with us and would I like to call and discuss. After talking to Paul, they came back with a better term sheet, which I asked my commercial lawyer Andrew Throssell to modify.

We agreed to a deal which wasn't the best for us upfront, but they are the world's biggest contact lens laboratory, with at least a 44% share of the world contact lens market. It could result in a royalty stream in several years' time. The agreement was sent to their attorney and Ed sent a proposed agreement to us. One paragraph in his proposal allowed J&J to give thirty-two days' notice to cancel the agreement and allow J&J to use the intellectual property without cost to them.

At time of writing, the original patent has only about ten years to run. J&J say it will take three to four years to get FDA approvals and go to the market. We have FDA approval for lathe-cut custom lenses and using $510k approval (or substantially equivalent) for cast moulding should be faster and more straightforward.

In my discussions with J&J the guy running the project told me that they had never cast moulded a lens that was truncated and had a front surface that included a slope, only lenses that have a spherical or toroidal surface.

From Jacksonville I flew to Atlanta, hired a car and drove to the Ciba facility, about 195km from the airport. At the meeting were eight people. I did my presentation, with someone placing a bifocal lens on his own eye. They spent most of the time finding fault with the lens. I showed the positive results from at least ten prominent doctors, but they were not convinced - or maybe this was their way to negotiate a favourable deal? One person present was their head of bifocal R&D, Dr Lindlaker, who has patents on a translating lens.

An Australian doctor I knew who was working in Ciba's R&D told me that at meetings held to discuss our lens, Lindlaker had dismissed our lens outright, even though all the translating lenses made to his designs did not work. He told me that Ciba has made many attempts to get the lens to work and concluded that: "a soft translating lens just won't work." At meetings held to discuss the samples of the cast moulded lenses I had sent, the doctor told me Lindlaker hadn't even looked at our lens and was totally negative about them.

After the meeting I had coffee with Ciba's deal maker, Lynn Winterton. He was very nice and said that although the lens had faults, maybe they could come up with something.

Within a week he sent me the following email:

> 10/10/2011
>
> Don
>
> Thanks for taking the time & for making a concerted effort to visit us.
>
> In reviewing the opportunities, we still believe that your design(s) will suffer from unacceptable clinical comfort-issues; much like they exhibit now. Like we indicated, in our discussions, we do not see how one will avoid the 'parting line' discomfort issues your current lens designs experience. Removing this parting line will involve novel designs, novel manufacturing approaches and a concerted effort; not merely tweaking your current designs.
>
> We think that there may be a possibility of collaboration which may bring about a novel lens design that may work, although at this juncture that is speculation. From our perspective, such a collaboration might begin by our first licensing (or acquiring) your patents in this arena, which would then allow us to move forward with a novel design for a translating lens. To this end, have you put a dollar-figure on your current IP from which we could begin negotiations? This discussion may also include a separate consultation agreement, for yourself, working with us on such a project.
>
> Please let me know your candid thoughts.
>
> Kind Regards, Lynn

I replied that I would get back to him.

Turned out Ciba (Novartis) had just acquired Alcon from Nestle and nobody was able to make any decisions - including the guy we were negotiating with.

After Atlanta came Bausch and Lomb in Rochester. Joe Barr, who was Professor of Optometry in Ohio State University and editor of Contact Lens Spectrum, was vice president. An Australian optometrist, Ian Cox, was head of their R&D and was also present at the meeting. They tried the lenses on and were amazed that they translated; no mention at all of any comfort problem. They both kept asking me if the lenses were moulded. I showed them the moulded shells I had with me that clearly showed the bifocal impression. I left lenses with them and they later copied the results of their examination of the lenses, which were very positive. Joe subsequently emailed me that such a lens was not a priority for them at this time but if it was up to him, it would be a no-brainer. An investment group owns them and the talk is that they will probably be sold when the market improves. It wasn't easy doing anything with large companies, as getting a result has to pass through many people all protecting their jobs.

London and the Ida Mann Plaque

When we returned from London in 1971, we had lived in Dalkeith, in the same suburb as Professor Dame Ida Mann. I often called to visit her, and on one visit I mentioned that the annual meeting of the Australian Contact Lens Society was to be held in Perth, and that I was presenting a paper. She asked when I would be speaking and she, together with visiting world-renowned UK ophthalmologist Dorothy Parker, came to the meeting. Before delivering my paper I introduced both Ida and Dorothy to the members and said how honoured we all were that they had attended. At the time ophthalmologists were forbidden to speak or attend meetings with optometrists, but Ida was so well respected that the ophthalmologist establishment did not say anything.

A young optometrist from Melbourne, Brien Holden, was at the meeting. He told me that it was worthwhile coming to Perth just to hear my paper. Brien was to become one of the world's most prominent and major players in the advancement of contact lenses.

In September 2012 we travelled to London, where I was invited to unveil the Blue Plaque at the London home of Professor Dame Ida Mann. It was great.

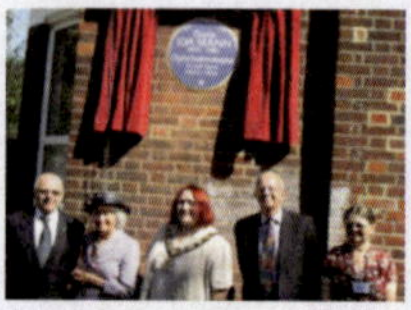

Don Ezekiel (left) unveiling an English Heritage Blue Plaque on 5th September 2012, in Kilburn, London, at the location of the place of residence from 1902–1934 of Professor Dame Ida Mann. Pictured are the speakers at the event, optometrist Donald Ezekiel from Perth Australia, Ida Mann's niece, Jill Mann, Mayor of Camden, councillor Heather Johnson, Professor Roger Buckley and Margaret Pelling of English Heritage. Also at the unveiling was the instigator of the event, contact lens historian and author Tim Bowden and Moorfields head of optometry, Dan Ehrlich.

This article appeared in *Home News and Features.*

New Plaque for Contact Lens Pioneer

A contact lens pioneer and the first woman consultant at Moorfields has been honoured with an English Heritage commemorative plaque on her former house in London. Dame Ida Mann helped introduce the slit lamp into the UK in 1921. She also brought world contact lens leader Josef Dallos and pioneer George Nissel over to the UK.

In 1937 she helped set up the first contact lens clinic at Cavendish Square, London and Moorfields contact lens department.

Dame Ida Mann also worked on mustard gas keratitis and wrote a book which was the definitive text for over 40 years on the development of the eye in embryo. She started a new life in Australia in 1949, conducting much ground-breaking work on trachoma among the indigenous Australians. She was still working when she died in 1983.

The house in which Dame Ida lived between 1902 and 1934 is at 13 Minster Road … however, due to the nature of the property's corner site, the plaque actually sits on a wall beneath the street sign for Fordwych Road. Fortuitously, this is the street in which Ida was born in 1893. Ida Mann was remarkable in so many ways. From 1914 she trained at the London Hospital for Women in Judd Street, near where the RNIB is now located. She moved to St. Mary's Hospital in 1917 as soon as that institution began educating women and, on qualifying, applied for every job she saw on the notice board. The one she got was that of ophthalmic house surgeon and her supervisor encouraged her to consider specialising in the eye from that moment, on the basis that this subject would be 'suitable for a girl'. An accomplished anatomist, she went on to produce the standard work on ocular embryology, making best use of perhaps the finest collection of embryos in any hospital at the time. She was instrumental in introducing the slit lamp to the UK in 1921 and in travelling to Budapest in 1937 to persuade Dr Josef Dallos, the pioneering contact lens practitioner, to come to Britain. She would go on to be the first president of the Contact Lens Society in 1946. She was the first woman professor of ophthalmology and the first woman professor (in any subject) at the University of Oxford.

> Then in the 1940s she emigrated to Australia and began a whole second career specialising in trachoma among Aboriginal communities, thereby pioneering the concept of geographical ophthalmology. Still working to the end, she died while writing at her desk.
>
> Just as I have given a highly condensed account above, it would be impossible to summarise such a long, varied and prestigious career on a plaque. Professor Roger Buckley, an eye surgeon and Honorary Fellow of the College of Optometrists nonetheless made a valiant attempt in his opening address in the presence of the Mayor of Camden, when he referred to it as a 'headlong dash' of a career. English Heritage, however, have gone to the opposite extreme and simply written 'ophthalmologist' on the plaque. What this conceals is perhaps one of her most lasting legacies.
>
> Ida Mann was one of the first ophthalmologists to pay proper respect to optometrists as professional equals a point which the distinguished Australian optometrist Don Ezekiel made at the unveiling before pulling the cord. The Contact Lens Society was the first inter-professional group of its type and a forerunner of the multi-disciplinary BCLA. The committee under her was composed so that every role, including those of secretary and treasurer, was held jointly by an ophthalmologist and an optometrist.
>
> The unveiling of the plaque marked the culmination of a campaign by Tim Bowden, begun in 2005. Tim is also the special adviser on the history of contact lenses to our College museum. The ceremony was disrupted by a faulty microphone, an overhead aircraft and a lorry delivering a skip, but despite this the event passed very successfully in brilliant sunshine. Don Ezekiel travelled 14,500 miles from Perth to see Kilburn's latest memorial, so I suggest that you bear that in mind if you find yourself in the area and make the considerably smaller effort to go and look.

After the unveiling we went to Ashford in Kent to attend the 2012 Congress of the ISCLS. I read a paper on the bifocal lens and was made an Honorary Life Member of the Society. It is a small exclusive group with the world's best contact lens practitioners as members. Very nice being honoured by this prestigious group.

Budapest and Prague

From England we flew to Budapest, where our friends Malcolm and Francis Steinberg joined us. We spent a few days there, which was lovely, and then on a boat cruise down the Danube via Vienna, calling in to several other towns to Nuremberg. Then we travelled by bus to the beautiful city of Prague for a few days. The hotel was lovely and we stayed close to the main square, just a few minutes' walk from the Jewish quarter. We had been to Prague before on our 1963 honeymoon travels, but had stayed further out from the city centre.

Malcolm and I took a bus trip to Tretzin (Theresienstadt) where my grandparents were sent. My grandmother (my mother's mother) perished there. My grandfather was sent from Theresienstadt to Auschwitz, where he also perished.

On a tour of Prague we were taken by bus to a beautiful hilltop castle on the other side of the river. How the people lived in the old days! After the tour Challis wanted some water and Malcolm and I misunderstood this and thought the girls were going to the toilet. Malcolm and I waited outside the toilets for some time and when the girls did not appear we walked to the corner where the bus had dropped us off. No sign of the girls. Malcolm stayed at the bus stop while I went back to see if I could find our wives. No luck in finding them so I returned to the bus stop. No Malcolm, no wives and no bus.

I asked a young student at a tram stop how to get to the main square and he took me there by tram and by train. On both the bus and train I asked my new friend where I needed to pay. He told me not to worry as it was lunch time and no inspectors would be about. When I got to the hotel Challis just said, "What took you so long!"

We then went to Israel for seven days, flying Czech Airlines. Our travel agent booked us business class, as it only cost an extra $25. Business class was exactly the same as economy, except the centre seat was empty!

Olivia's Bat Mitzvah

Olivia's bat mitzvah was held in Israel on Saturday 27 September 2013. Sasha and her family and Paul and Tanya joined us at the Kabbalah centre in Tel Aviv. It was lovely. Russell was included by carrying the Torah when the ark was closed. Paul opened and closed the ark and I carried the Torah from the ark and returned it to the ark. Lunch downstairs at the centre was lovely. They are a caring inclusive group and Rivka commented that it was so nice to see the congregation being happy.

Mordechai (Motke) Adler, Rivka's partner in Israel, was a religious Jew before he experienced three concentration camps. He has not believed in religion or been to a synagogue since. He came to the service and thoroughly enjoyed it. It was wonderful to see the family, they are so very nice. Motke wrote a book on his life in the extermination camps and life afterwards in Israel. He gave me a copy in Hebrew but many attempts to have it translated into English in Perth were not successful. Mokte had it translated into English and gave me a copy when we were in Israel. I could not put it down and was quite moved and even depressed reading it. How someone could go through this I cannot imagine. He is such a nice person and I am fortunate to have met and spent some time with him. I do hope that it is published and widely read. It's the most moving account I have read on the Holocaust.

We were both happy that Paul and Tanya were included in the Kabbalah congregation. Paul hired a car and with Malcolm and Tanya drove us to Jerusalem on the Sunday where we visited the Holocaust Memorial, Vad Vashem. We only had two hours there as it closed early for Succoth. We could have stayed there a full day. I must go back one day and see it properly.

Israel was hot but is an interesting country. The family makes it special. When the family returned home I asked Olivia what the best part of her travels was. She replied, "Being with my cousins." Lovely.

From Israel we flew to Istanbul, where we stayed at the Orient Express Hotel. The hotel staff were very nice. We enjoyed Istanbul and hope to get back there again.

Sasha and her family also followed to Istanbul, as did Paul and Tanya. They stayed in the new part of the city, over the Bosphorus Strait, while we stayed in the old part of the city.

One night Paul suggested we join them at a recommended

restaurant on the square in the new part of Istanbul. We caught a taxi and were dropped at the large square, which was surrounded by upmarket shops. The restaurant turned out to be at the other end of the square. As we walked up the square a large crowd of demonstrators came towards us. We walked to the side of the demonstrators, but Challis saw that the restaurant was on the opposite side of the square. I took her hand and we walked through the demonstrators. No problem - but no Paul at the restaurant. Challis went inside to a table while I waited outside for Paul. Still no Paul. Challis said we eat or we leave. We had a lovely meal but still no Paul.

Outside the restaurant police in protective gear with shields and water cannons were assembled. Great! This should be interesting! Challis suggested we get out of there before we got caught up in a riot. We left, and shortly after there was a riot. We caught a taxi to the hotel and were greeted by the hotel staff telling us our family had been frantically calling to see if we were okay. Paul and Tanya saw there was trouble and went back to their hotel.

CHAPTER FIFTEEN

JOHNSON & JOHNSON

The Agreement with J&J

When the lab was sold we retained all patents on the soft translating bifocal lens. Fortunately, Masel did not see any value in the bifocal lens and only saw their ongoing costs with patents. He felt that the lens was so different to all other bifocal lenses that it would be difficult to market.

I was still trying to get one of the large labs to take the lens on. It had been sixteen months since I visited J&J. I had come to an agreement with their dealmaker Ed Rastelli, but it took a further four months to get through J&J's legal section.

On February 6th, 2013, the agreement with J&J was signed off. Paul was terrific. He had found a great attorney in Henry Ward III, who with Paul managed to get the deal done. We didn't get much upfront, but I think J&J will work it aggressively, as they could see it would give them a huge market opportunity. They estimated the actual current bifocal market sales then to be worth $200 million dollars with current lens designs.

The patents have a limited time span, but there are also patents pending on the manufacturing process, which if granted will be extended for the life of the patent - a further twenty-one years. I won't be around but Paul and Sasha may benefit from the royalties, which could be substantial.

During our negotiations with J&J, Ed Restalli sent the following email:

> 26 January 2013
>
> One point that I would like to make is that, as you know, the current presbyopic lens market is fickle in that there quite a few products out on the market, the majority of them with modest worldwide sales. This is because the products don't meet the needs of a broad presbyopic market. We have two presbyopic products on the market and will continue to work

> in the space and maintain presbyopic products that make sense financially and from an Acuvue portfolio perspective. Even though the two products we have enjoy only modest sales, we continue to carry them as they have a place in the portfolio.

Later that year I spoke with my contacts at J&J, Hussain and Greg Hofman. They were going to come to Perth to get the technology transfer, but the moulded lenses and inserts I sent has given them all they need. We made the inserts in two parts; one with the back surface with truncation and one with the lens powers. This allowed us to change the powers and use the same piece for the back surface with truncation. J&J were making the insert in one piece. It took them some time to do this, as until then they had only lathed standard spheres and toric lenses and the bifocal is a more complex design. Their lathing of an insert took them thirteen hours! They hadn't got the edge smooth enough, but I was hopeful they would do it very well.

Jacksonville

Whenever I was in New York I visited J&J in Jacksonville. On one occasion, the 6pm flight back from Jacksonville was cancelled due to mechanical problems. The replacement flight was rescheduled to leave at midnight and arrived in JFK airport at three am. When we arrived the airport was deserted, apart from the cleaners. The passengers from my flight milled around the deserted taxi stand. A taxi arrived and the guy ahead of me hopped in. I asked the driver if he could order a taxi for me. He asked where I was going (Manhattan) and he told me to hop in. I sat in the front seat. The driver was from Eastern Europe and built like he could look after himself. The passenger in the back was a big black guy who started to argue with the driver, saying that as there were now two passengers the fare should be less. The driver told him in no certain way to pay the full price or to get out. He agreed to pay and asked if he would take Visa. No - only cash. The taxi stopped in the Bronx at a 7-11 shop and he went to get cash for the fare. I was concerned that the black guy would return with his mates and shoot the taxi driver. While we were waiting two police cars tore past. I asked where they were headed. Taxi guy said there was a housing estate nearby. "Bad news. Shootings. Drugs. Don't go there." The guy came back, paid the amount asked for and I was driven to my hotel. Next day the TV news reported a fatal shooting at the housing complex in the Bronx at three-thirty am. Paul and Tanya both said: *"No-one goes to the Bronx, and especially not at three-thirty in the morning!"*

That Christmas Paul, Tanya and eight-month-old Zahara came from New York to spend two weeks with us in Perth. Challis and I loved having them stay. Zahara was just lovely and a very good baby. Twelve hours sleep a night. We enjoyed playing with her and watching her at her swimming lessons. Seeing Sasha, Russell, Livy and Max love her was something we will treasure. So nice and special for us all to have the opportunity to share this part of her growing up. Olivia and Max just loved her and Zahara reciprocated. Just lovely to see. When seeing them off at the airport Zahara clung to Olivia. They will all miss her.

Profile in Clinical and Experimental Optometry

In 2014, Nathan Efron called and told me he wanted to write an article about me, but would prefer it be a profile, rather than an obituary! He published a wonderful article, which appeared *Clinical and Experimental Optometry*. The full version is in the Appendix.

CHAPTER SIXTEEN

INTERNATIONAL AWARD OF EXCELLENCE

Global Specialty Contact Lens Symposium Award of Excellence

I received from Craig W. Norman, Director of the Vision Research Institute at Michigan College of Optometry, Ferris State University the following email.

> September 5th, 2014
>
> Dear Don,
>
> Congratulations! On behalf of the Global Specialty Lens Symposium Education Committee it is my pleasure to inform you that the 2015 GSLS Award of Excellence will be presented to you and other scleral lens pioneers in recognition of your years of outstanding contributions to the world of contact lenses. A plaque is little reward for the larger-than-life impact you have had on vision care, but we would love to present this award to you on January 22 during the opening session of the 2015 conference.
>
> The award is given annually to one or more distinguished clinician, scholar and/or scientist to recognise their lifelong achievements in the field of contact lenses, especially as they relate to specialty contact lenses. The individuals selected are those being recognised for their career's contribution to the field of contact lenses, including development, practice, translation of knowledge and education, and scholarly activity, all of which moved the field of contact lenses forward in seminal ways. Your work in the scleral lens field definitely falls into this category.
>
> You will be joining other distinguished winners of this award as Dr. Donald Korb and Professor Brien Holden were previous honourees in 2014 and 2013 respectively.
>
> We hope you can join us for the award ceremonies.
>
> Best regards, Craig

This is the first time I had been acknowledged by my profession and, given the previous awardees were Donald Korb (who I believe is the very best optometrist and researcher) and prominent contact lens researcher Brien Holden, it is the best compliment I could have.

Challis couldn't come as she was scheduled to have another back operation. Sasha came with me and we stayed in Las Vegas for four nights. The meeting was great and the presentation of the award – an engraved glass piece - was really lovely. Many people introduced themselves and asked to be photographed with me. One doctor told me that he had fitted his first five patients and that I had changed his life. Very nice.

Sasha put this note on Facebook, which received lots of comments.

> "Hi all, Don's presentation was really lovely and he was introduced as the man who epitomises the word 'pioneer' in the CL industry. He spoke really well and all sorts of people are lining up to shake his hand."

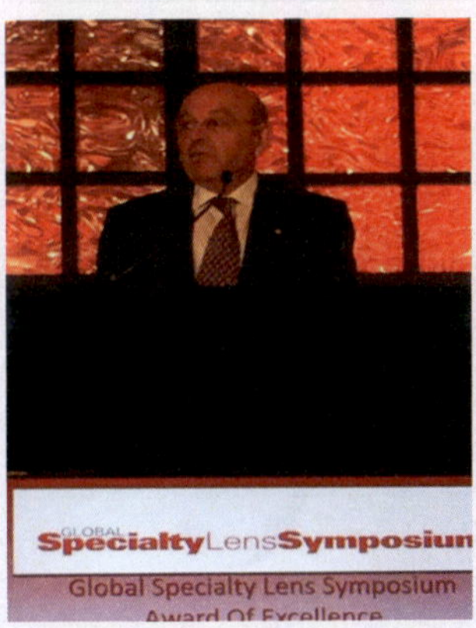

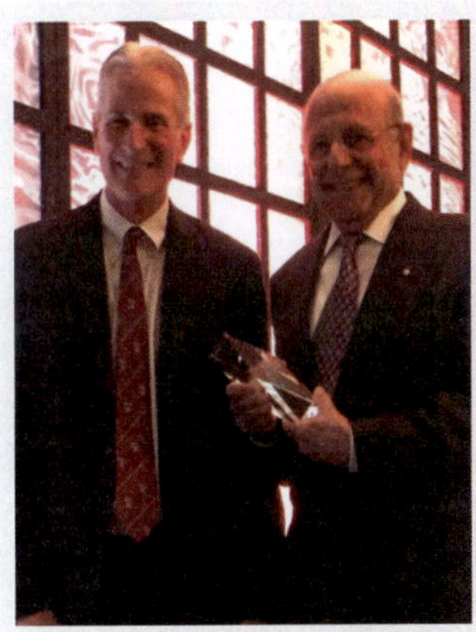

Don Ezekiel addresses the symposium with Dr Ed Bennett from the Global Specialty Lens Symposium education committee.

Don Ezekiel, right, receives his award from Dr Ed Bennett, a member of the Global Specialty Lens Symposium education committee.

This was Ed's introduction:

> The GSLS Award of Excellence is given annually to distinguished clinicians, scholars and scientists to recognise their lifelong achievements in the field of contact lenses, especially as they relate to specialty contact lenses. Mr Ezekiel an innovative contact lens practitioner and manufacturer, was a leader in the contact lens industry for more than 40 years and in 1997 was made a Member of the Order of Australia in recognition of service to the optometric profession and to the development of scleral contact lenses.

This report came out following the symposium:

> Contact lens innovator Don Ezekiel from Western Australia has been honoured as a scleral lens pioneer at the 2015 Global Specialty Lens Symposium in the USA.
>
> Three others who also received scleral lens pioneer awards at the symposium this year were Ken Pullum from the United Kingdom, Rients Visser from The Netherlands and American ophthalmologist Perry Rosenthal who described Mr Ezekiel as "the grandfather of gas permeable scleral lenses."
>
> Mr Ezekiel's daughter Sasha, who attended the ceremony, said her father was introduced as 'the man who epitomises the word pioneer in the contact lens industry.'
>
> Mr Ezekiel told Australian Optometry: 'When I presented a paper on the gas permeable lens in 1983 at the annual meeting of the BCLA in Harrogate, the write up in the optical press was that no-one believed the results I showed of forty-three patients wearing the lens. It was the first time RGP scleral lens fitting had been described. It was most satisfying that some 80 per cent of papers at the recent GSLS meeting were on GP scleral lenses.'
>
> Mr Ezekiel graduated in optometry in 1957 and later went to Sydney to be taught scleral lens fitting by Lloyd Hewitt. In 1963 he travelled to London to complete an advanced contact lens degree before returning to Perth to work in the family practice founded by his father Elias and uncle Abraham.

```
Mr Ezekiel established his own practice in Perth in
1970 specialising in contact lenses and as he couldn't
source the contact lenses he wanted, began designing
and making them for his patients.

He started his own contact lens manufacturing company,
Western Australian Contact Lens Manufacturing, later
renamed Gelflex Laboratories. He sold the company four
years ago and is semi-retired but still does some
consulting.
```

CHAPTER SEVENTEEN

FAMILY CONTINUED

In February 2016 I again got stuck in Jacksonville when visiting Johnson & Johnson. The six pm flight to New York was cancelled due to bad weather. The hotel at the airport was fully booked and the only option seemed to be to bed down on couches in the airport lounge. Paul called and told me he had booked me into a motel nearby. It was like being in 1960 movie! Basic and cheap, but at least I had a shower.

Birth of Zed

I caught the six am flight to New York and arrived in time for the birth of Paul and Tanya's son. Challis and I were both there.

According to Kabbalah ritual, the night before the bris men would meet to discuss the significance of the bris. It started at about eleven pm and guys came and went. Around twelve thirty am Benjamin - the head teacher at Kabbalah - started telling jokes. He was very good and enjoyable. We left at one thirty am.

The bris was nice and I streamed it live to Sasha and family in Perth. The baby's name was announced as Joseph. I said to Paul that this was a nice name (we had been concerned that it might be a *very different name*!) He told us firmly that Joseph was not his name, his name was Zed. Classic Paul. I had told the Perth family on Skype that the baby's name was Joseph, and had to call back and correct myself.

Max's Bar Mitzvah

In 2016 Sasha's son Max had his bar mitzvah at Temple David in Perth. He read his portion well and we were all proud of him. Paul came from New York and Eric's son Ron came from Israel, so it was very special.

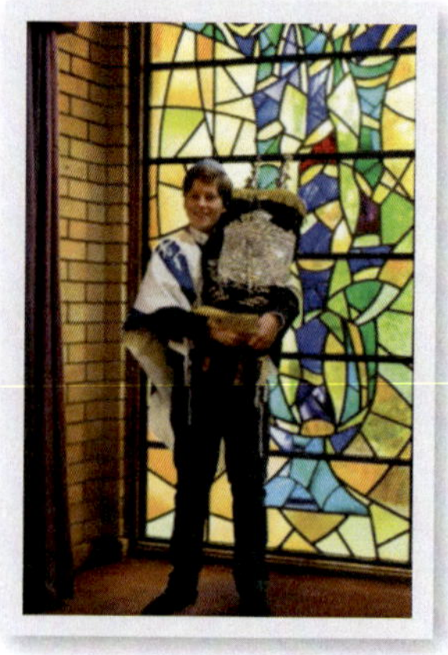

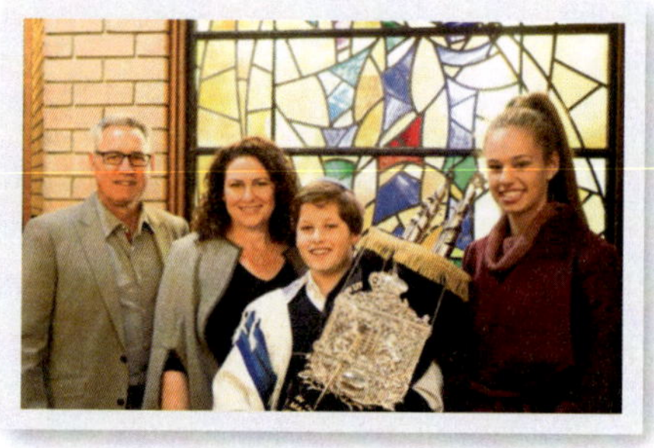

Turning Eighty

Malcolm Steinberg, Les Edelman and I started a group of old Jewish guys we call the 'Ulta Kuckers'. We had lunch at different restaurants every two weeks. There were seventeen in the group, with ten to fifteen regularly attending the lunch.

Les told me about a concert being planned by Jewish folk who were turning eighty, and that I should join. I had already reached that milestone, but he told the review arranger, Judy Freedman, that I was interested in joining. Judy wrote and arranged the music, directed and produced the show. It was to be held four months later, in September. Rehearsals were fun and enjoyable. One good thing about the rehearsals was getting to see and to know folk again who I had only spoke to in passing over the years.

The concert was on Sunday September 3rd, 2017. There was a sell-out crowd with a waiting list. I suggested we present an 'Oscar' to Judy Freedman, and the group thought that was a good idea and that I should present the award. I needed a good story so I asked Paul for help. He suggested that I call Benjamin at the Kabbala centre in New York, as he had a large repertoire of jokes and stories. I called him and used one of his stories in my presentation.

> A group of forty-year-olds decide to have a reunion. Where do we go? Let's go to Goldberg's restaurant. Waitresses are well endowed; they all have great bodies and are gorgeous.
>
> 50-year reunion. Where do we go? Let's go to Goldberg's restaurant. Good food and nice environment.
>
> 60-year reunion. Where do we go? Let's go to Goldberg's restaurant. Music not too loud. Can hear each other and the food is decent.
>
> 70-year reunion. Where do we go? Let's go to Goldberg's restaurant. Close by with easy access and the bathroom is near the restaurant.
>
> 80-year reunion. Where do we go? Let's go to Goldberg's restaurant. Good idea - we haven't been there before!!

And speaking of Goldberg, I met him last week. Asked him how he was. Great, he said I am getting married tomorrow. So who is the lucky lady? An amazingly beautiful twenty-five-year-old with a body to die for.

Goldberg, Goldberg, Goldberg. You are ninety-six. She is twenty-five with a body to die for. Could this be not ideal for one's health?

I know, I know ... but if she dies, she dies!

An article in *The Maccabean* (Perth's Jewish newspaper) reported the show was enjoyed by all. We had fun putting it on.

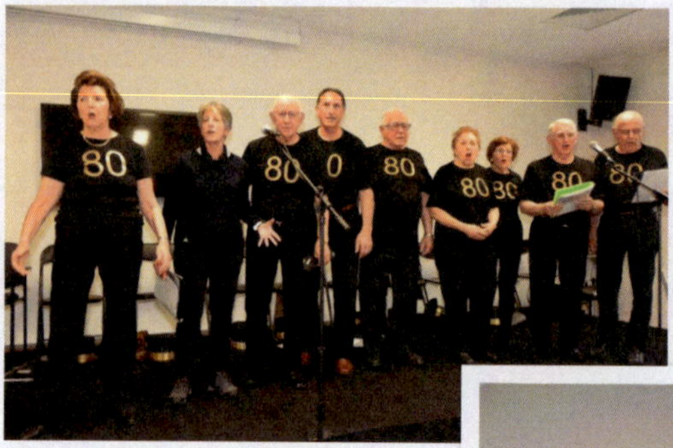

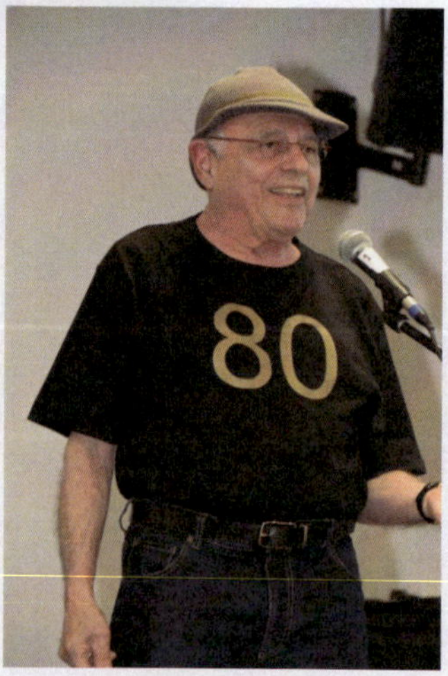

CHAPTER EIGHTEEN
CONTACT LENS AND OPTICAL COLLECTION

Phillip Beilby

The pathology lecturer in my optometry course, ophthalmologist Ken Bardon-Brown, had worked with Dallos, from whom he learned his glass scleral lens fitting procedure. Ken practised in Perth, fitting glass scleral lenses, but had problems getting his lens, which he ordered from Dallos in London, as they took three months to arrive from London.

Ken explained this predicament to Phillip Beilby, a motor mechanic and a patient of his. Phillip had developed trachoma, an eye problem resulting in the scarring of his corneas. Ken asked Phillip if he could make glass scleral lenses for him, to save waiting so long having them sent from London. Apart from being a scleral lenses patient, Phillip knew nothing about scleral lenses, let alone how they were made. He mastered the technology from textbooks and made a scleral glass manufacturing bench from bits and pieces, including a motor from an old washing machine. This allowed him to make excellent lenses. Ken died at a young age, and Phillip took over the fitting of the scleral lenses for his patients. As he was the only one at the time in Perth fitting scleral lenses (and a motor mechanic by trade!) State Parliament passed a law allowing him to fit scleral lenses. When he retired, Phillip passed his patients on to me.

Phillip was a lovely man. His poor vision had not prevented him from enlisting in the army during the war, and he was sent to Singapore. When Singapore fell he was captured and sent on a ship to Japan to work in the coal mines. The ship was torpedoed by an American submarine and he spent three days in an oil slick, which he says saved his life from being eaten by sharks before being rescued by an US submarine, the *Pampanpanto,* which is now in the Maritime Museum in San Francisco. Phillip contributed a chapter on his war time experience in a book, and kindly gave me a copy. He played the clarinet and saxophone in Ron Jenkins' band, a very popular band in the fifties and sixties.

I visited Phillip often and complimented him on his work. I asked him if I could purchase his glass work bench when he retired. He didn't forget, and called one day to tell me he was retiring. He gave me his wonderful glass scleral manufacturing bench, together with a large collection of glass scleral lenses, which I added to my antique optical collection.

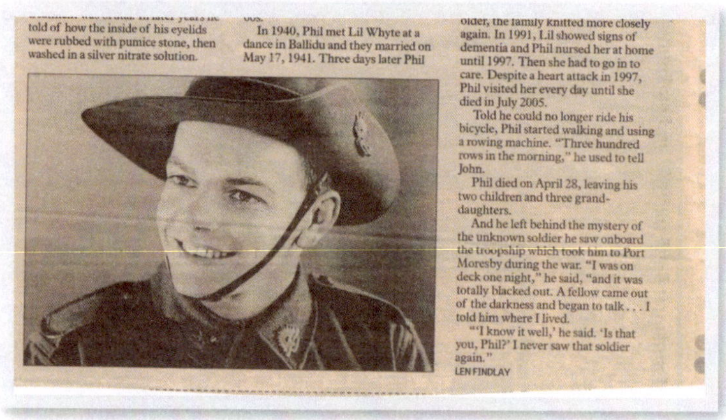

told of how the inside of his eyelids were rubbed with pumice stone, then washed in a silver nitrate solution.

In 1940, Phil met Lil Whyte at a dance in Ballidu and they married on May 17, 1941. Three days later Phil

older, the family knitted more closely again. In 1991, Lil showed signs of dementia and Phil nursed her at home until 1997. Then she had to go in to care. Despite a heart attack in 1997, Phil visited her every day until she died in July 2005.

Told he could no longer ride his bicycle, Phil started walking and using a rowing machine. "Three hundred rows in the morning," he used to tell John.

Phil died on April 28, leaving his two children and three grand-daughters.

And he left behind the mystery of the unknown soldier he saw onboard the troopship which took him to Port Moresby during the war. "I was on deck one night," he said, "and it was totally blacked out. A fellow came out of the darkness and began to talk . . . I told him where I lived.

"'I know it well,' he said. 'Is that you, Phil?' I never saw that soldier again."

LEN FINDLAY

Article about Phillip Beilby in the West Australian.

Whenever I visited contact lens practitioners for the laboratory, I would tell them of my interest in collecting interesting old contact lenses and they often showed me what they had in their bottom drawer. I added some wonderful lenses and unwanted fitting sets for my collection. Part of the collection was displayed in my practice but when Damon took it over, I took the collection with me. The big question was, what would I do with it?

Patrick Caroline and the Contact Lens Museum

An optometrist friend Mark Lucy made an Apple photo book showing pieces from my antique optical and contact lens collection, and at meetings and conferences I asked around trying to find a home for them. Australian universities were interested but would only catalogue and store the collection, as they had nowhere to display it.

I wanted it to be displayed so the pieces wouldn't be forgotten.

At a meeting in Las Vegas I showed the catalogue to Pat Caroline from Pacific University in Portland USA. He became excited and asked what I wanted for the collection. Nothing, I told him. Just that it be displayed, plus plane tickets for Challis and me to visit it.

Pat visited Perth and we went through the pieces. I had saved all the correspondence I had ever received during the early days of soft contact lenses, including the first soft lenses made by Sfofa Czechoslovakia still in their original vials. I had also kept invoices, practitioner fitting and patient handling notes, plus the scleral work bench from Phillip Beilby and many fitting sets and glass lenses.

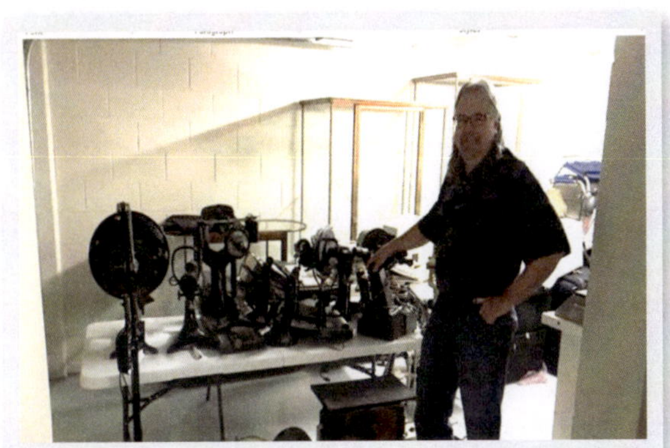

Pat looking through the collection in the garage in Wellington Street.

The number of times Pat said, "Oh my God!" when going through the collection and correspondence was amazing. Everything was shipped to Portland, including Phillip's bench and Ida Mann's scleral fitting set, which Pat was very excited to have and carried home with him. It became part of the Contact Lens Museum.

Part of the collection was subsequently displayed at the Global Lens Symposium meeting in Las Vegas in 2018.

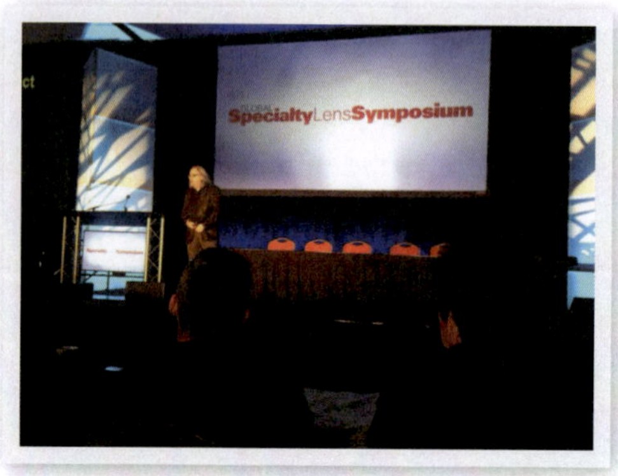

Pat in Las Vegas.

An article from *Contact Lens Spectrum*, April 2018.

> The much-anticipated premier of the Contact Lens Museum occurred in the 2018 GSLS Exhibit Hall. The brainchild of Patrick Caroline, in collaboration with scleral lens pioneer Donald Ezekiel, Dip Opt (WA), and Craig Norman, many of the early scleral contact lenses as well as contact lens equipment, instrumentation, education materials, and other items were on display.

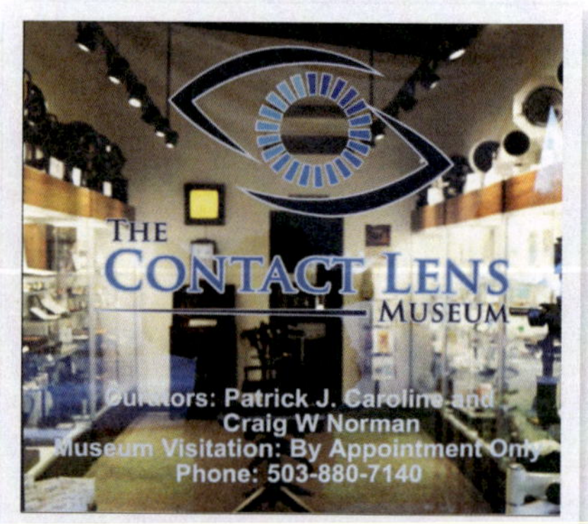

Contact Lens Museum Opens

I flew to Portland, Oregon, where Pat Caroline and Craig Norman, the curators of the museum, picked me up. We all stayed at Pat's home for the night. He collects antique juke boxes and gramophones, all restored and in working condition. Amazing. Pat's wife Jiah is lovely, she made us feel very welcome.

The opening of the museum was very nice. Pat and I cut the ribbon. Pat and Jiah have done a wonderful job. I am on the museum board, together with Pat, Craig, Joe Barr and Roy Wesley, son of Newton Wesley, the founder of the Wesley and Jesson laboratory. Roy is donating his father's pieces to the museum. I think larger premises will be needed!

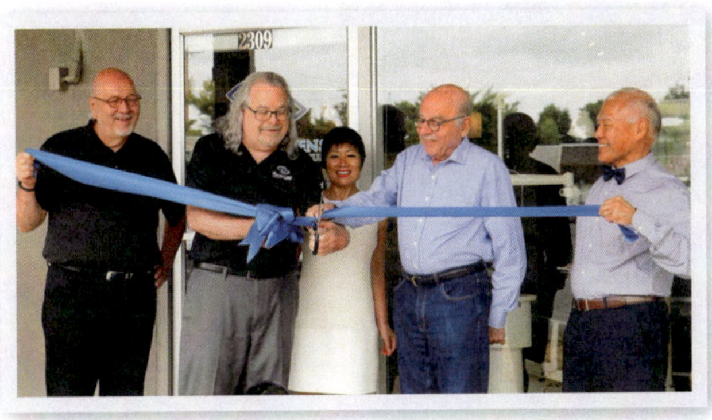

Opening of Museum. Craig Norman, Pat Caroline, Zia, me and Roy Wesley. Craig Norman and Pat Caroline are the people responsible for the museum.

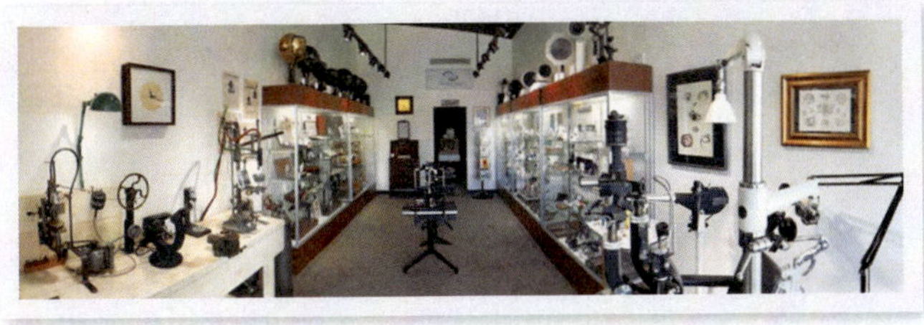

Some of the instruments and lenses I donated on display.

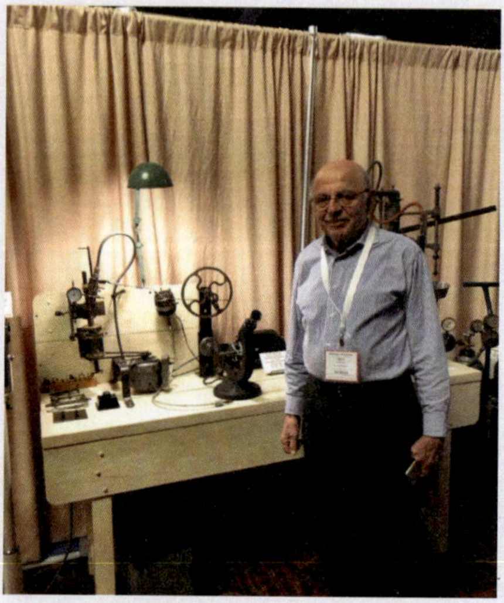

Glass scleral manufacturing work bench made by Phillip Beilby, the only glass moulding work bench in the world in working order.

I am on the board of the museum, and in 2023 I attended, via Zoom, the annual meeting. The museum is progressing and expanding by including ophthalmology and spectacle antiques. Pat Caroline's presentation on the current and possible future position of the museum was enlightening.

During the Global Lens Symposium meeting in Las Vegas, Jason Nichols OD, MPH, PhD and editor of *Contact Lens Spectrum,* moderated a lively session as industry executives discussed their views on the present state of the contact lens market. I wrote this quote down from Jason (the italics are mine):

> "The global contact lens market today is estimated to be worth anywhere from \$1.3/1.5 billion per annum to … priceless. But the multifocal lens sales make up only 15% of the market - around \$200 million per annum."

I managed to stay seated! The market is clearly there and wanting a decent lens. I spoke to the guys on the J&J stand and told them that I thought something good was in the pipeline. They replied it was needed.

CHAPTER NINETEEN
THE END OF J&J AGREEMENT

Until now, I had been speaking with J&J at least every two weeks. Now my requests to speak with them were put off as they were 'collating the results', 'on holidays', or some other reason. I was sure something was up, as they had told me they had to decide by mid-February 2017 if they wanted to continue with the lens project. An extension required J&J to pay me US $500,000 for a one year extension, or US $750,000 for a two-year extension.

In November 2017 Tom Baugh, a US colleague, suggested I check on US patent application number 20130258274, titled 'Method and apparatus for providing variations of lower lid support structures of a translating multifocal contact lens'. I checked and found one of the 'co-inventors' being the same Greg Hofman who headed the bifocal lens project and with whom I worked closely with, and to whom I passed on all the design and technology.

Their application had a lot of miss-direction (a term we use in magic). Buried in the application they described a lens similar to our lens, but described it as a round lens (non-truncated) with a 'slope' (we call it a ledge). We had made and evaluated the lens they described and found it did not work as well as the truncated lens. In my files the diagram is accompanied with links dated January 2004. This design of the round lens incorporating a ledge did not perform as well as our truncated lens version so the project was not pursued. The application clearly is to get around my patent. I forcefully queried J&J about their patent application and indicated that I was not impressed.

Our US attorney, Henry Ward, said not to be concerned as the same examiner who approved our patent would be inspecting their application, and he was sure it would not be approved.

I passed all my J&J correspondence to Henry and Paul. Henry thought it was their way to get out of the payments for extension of the exclusivity, and part of their negotiating strategy.

J&J had had four years to get the cast moulding right. We managed to do this in about eighteen months. Their high-end lathes did not have the tool clearance to clear the lens ledge, causing chatter marks on the ledge, so their orders for moulding inserts had to be ordered from an overseas source. It appears that J&J spent time redesigning the lens as a round lens with what they called a slope (our ledge) clearly to get around my patents and to avoid future royalties.

J&J told me on several occasions during my visits to them that they did not have the technology to make a lens that was truncated (not round) and included surfaces that were not spherical or toroidal bit irregular. Yet our small laboratory managed to make the inserts and to cast mould the lens, without any of the technical support J&J has.

The early lenses J&J made were uncomfortable to wear, so they changed the lens material to a different material - with discomfort again resulting. Are these highly paid professionals serious? If the basic design is not correct, a change in material will not help! It is basic and obvious.

In emails and on visits I stressed the area at the ledge needed to be refined to achieve patient comfort. None of my advice appeared to have been taken.

Although they are the largest contact lens manufacturer, and would be the best to market the lens, I had doubts and misgivings that - with their ability to protect their own design and position, and with their recent launch of a simultaneous vision bifocal lens - they would be enthusiastic enough about the translating lens to take it to market.

Could they be trusted, when they had already applied for a patent that tried to get around the two US patents we received?

By now, a Greg Williby had taken over the bifocal lens project from Greg Hofman, who I had initially worked with. I believe Williby was responsible for taking J&J's latest 'me too' simultaneous vision lens to market and became responsible for the translating lens project.

Shortly after my firm query re their patent application J&J arranged a phone conference call with me. Greg Williby and Carl Evans (J&J patent attorney) were on the call to advise me that the current agreement would be terminated by J&J, but they "would be interested in negotiating a new agreement." When I subsequently checked the re-negotiation of a new agreement with J&J's deal maker Ed Rastelli, he had not heard anything about this.

As there had been a connection problem during the phone call, they copied me their PowerPoint presentation to explain their reason of termination. It included diagrams of the lens, showing it as a round lens with a 'slope', and the comment that 'this did not translate' being the reason that they wished to terminate our agreement.

This was not the lens described in our patents and detailed in our agreement. The lens described in our agreement and in our patents is a *truncated* lens.

POWERPOINT PRESENTATION FROM J&J ADVISING OF DECISION TO TERMNATE AGREEMENT.

Update (25 AUG 2017)

- JJV Decision to Terminate Current • Agreement, per Article 7.1
  - JJV has obligation to pay minimum royalty payments ($50k) for fourth (2018) and fifth (2019) years
  - JJV has obligation for legal expense for IP until termination date (60 days following written notice)
- JJV open to new agreement discussions

Translating Optics - Clinical Update (CR-5878, CR-5938)

- JJV Decision to Terminate Current • Agreement, per Article 7.1
  - JJV has obligation to pay minimum royalty payments ($50k) for fourth (2018) and fifth (2019) years
  - JJV has obligation for legal expense for IP until termination date (60 days following written notice)
- JJV open to new agreement discussions

Translating Optics - Clinical Update (CR-5878, CR-593)

I was advised in the call that the resulting lens did not achieve good translation. Their comment in Patent 20190072785 was: 'employs features in designs resulting in certain trade-offs. Comfort versus the extent of translation.'

A round lens is easier to make. We had tried and evaluated this lens design without a truncation but found it to not be as good as the truncated lens, which is why we did not pursue the design.

Update (25 AUG 2017)

- JJV Decision to Terminate Current • Agreement, per Article 7.1
    - JJV has obligation to pay minimum royalty payments ($50k) for fourth (2018) and fifth (2019) years
    - JJV has obligation for legal expense for IP until termination date (60 days following written notice)
- JJV open to new agreement discussions

Translating Optics - Clinical Update (CR-5878, CR-5938)

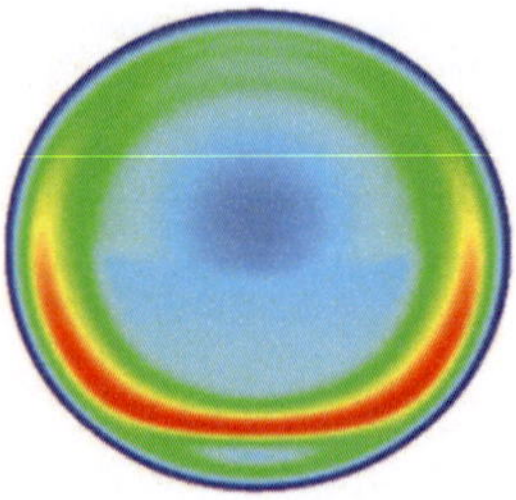

Two years earlier, in 2015, J&J had launched their new 1-day Acuvue Moist Multifocal Simultaneous vision bifocal lens (a variation of all simultaneous vision soft bifocal lenses available). At the time, I emailed Greg Hofman at J&J and asked him if their new 1-day Acuvue Moist Multifocal lens was any good. His reply follows:

```
Date: 11 February 2015

Hi Don,

We started the clinical trial yesterday. I am
currently processing the some of the data now. The
2015 product will be a new simultaneous vision
product. Translating lens is expected to be a large
improvement over this new product. That expectation
has been communicated to our board, so the "pressure"
is on, which is a good thing. Regards, Greg
```

And 13 Mar 2015:

```
Hi Don,
We have seen about ten subjects (25-30 total to be
completed) and we are observing quite good results.
No problems so far. The clinic is quite busy so I am
seeing only about two subjects a week; one is in the
clinic right now. We except to be completed in about
a month, but are nevertheless moving forward. We
have designed the optics and are hoping to make the
tools soon. We expect to make non-clinical lenses in
about a month to calibrate the tools and then move
on to making the clinical lenses. We likely will
alter the optics using the data from the ongoing
clinical trial. I just updated our stakeholders and
everyone seemed pleased. Best Regards, Greg
```

Many similar, positive emails were received. These are all recorded and I have them on file. As all communication with J&J to date had been positive, no Plan B had been contemplated. I contacted many cast moulding laboratories asking if there was any interest in the translating bifocal lens. All cast moulding labs have inventories of versions of the simultaneous vision bifocal lens and were not interested.

Some of the laboratories I contacted were Clerio, Coopervision, X-Cel, a Taiwanese lab, Andy Chrysilor, Bausch and Lomb, Alcon, Sauflon, Essilor, Menicon, and Specsavers.

Pat Caroline at Pacific University published articles describing the obvious advantages of a translating bifocal lens, and he had evaluated and loved the cast moulded Triton lenses we made. When I told him our agreement with J&J had been terminated and I was searching for options, he wrote to me.

```
Hello Don,

Your soft bifocal lens design has been a BIG topic
of conversation with our research team at Pacific
University. Is it possible for us to get our hands
on two or three of the lenses? We would like to
video the lenses on eye and get as much information
as we can to you before you start shopping it
```

around. Additionally, it might be helpful for you to say that the lens design is currently being evaluated at the Pacific University College of Optometry.

Needless-to-say, we can immediately get some state-of-the-art images to you, and we can serve as a resource to any company interested in licensing the design from you. Please feel free to use my name and that of Pacific University if you think it might be helpful.

Let me know how we might be able to get our hands on a few of the lenses. We are ready, willing and able to sign the necessary NDA and get cracking with the project and assist you in any way we can. It is clear that this design is probably going nowhere in the hands of J&J and the market truly does need an alternative to the current multifocal in the marketplace. All the best to you my friend, Pat.

We received another US patent on the bifocal lens. I saw that J&J were granted patents, with patent applications that had Jeffery Roffman, Greg Hofman and Khalid Chahab as 'inventors'. All have been in personal contact with me re the bifocal project. Greg Hofman, who I passed the technology to, and Khalid Chahab were both involved with the project, and Jeffery Roffman was their patent attorney. I have emails from them describing the progress of the project. They were all positive and advising the project was progressing well.

Unfortunately when Greg Williby took over the project he advised that he was starting the project over again.

CHAPTER TWENTY

MORE INTERNATIONAL RECOGNITION

Las Vegas: Global Contact Lens Symposium

The 2018 congress of the Global Contact Lens Symposium was held in Las Vegas from January 26th. I went there and back in less than a week. Pat Caroline spoke for an hour on the history of contact lenses. The Contact Lens Museum had a booth to promote the launch. Pat showed off many of my pieces and told everyone that they were from Don Ezekiel, "and if you see him, give him a big hug." Many did!

It was a very enjoyable meeting and it was good to catch up with people I knew, including Ivan Hare from Israel and Jim Marks from DAC, who came especially to see me.

US contact lens specialists Melissa Barnet and Lynette Johns had published a book titled *Contemporary Scleral Lenses Theory and Application.* They were more than pleased to see me and gave me a copy of the book, to which they each wrote a very nice comment on the front page.

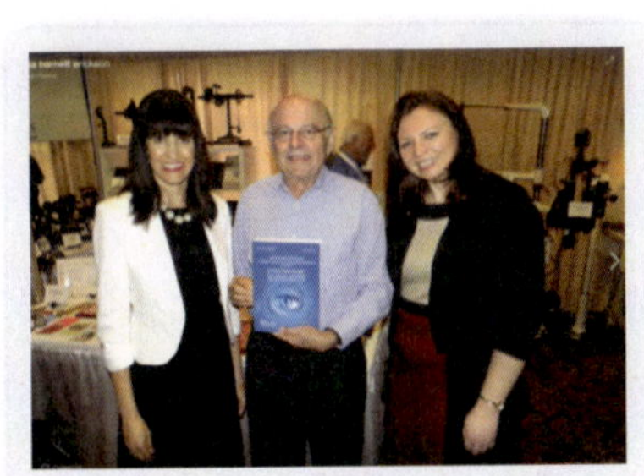

Melissa and Lynette presenting me a copy of their book.

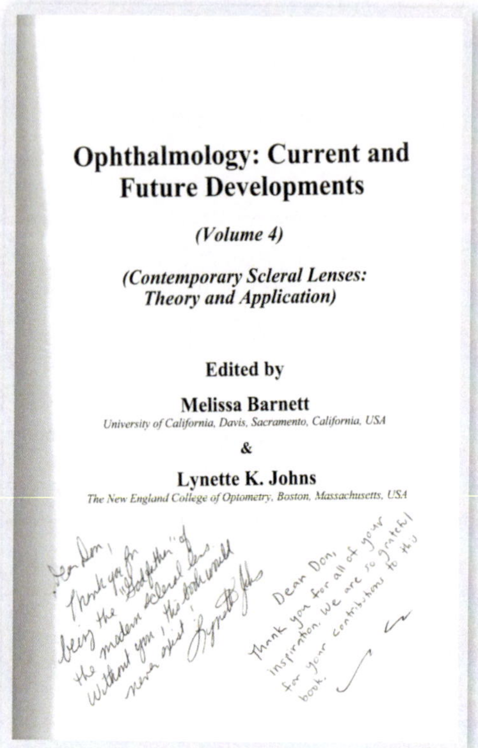

Ophthalmology: Current and Future Developments

(Volume 4)

(Contemporary Scleral Lenses: Theory and Application)

Edited by

Melissa Barnett
University of California, Davis, Sacramento, California, USA

&

Lynette K. Johns
The New England College of Optometry, Boston, Massachusetts, USA

Dear Don, Thank you for being the "Godfather" of the modern scleral lens. Without you, this book would never exist! Lynette Johns

Dear Don, Thank you for all of your inspiration. We are so grateful for your contributions to this book.

Melissa and Lynette's comments in the front page.

Daddi Fadel invited me to the Italian scleral lens conference and later joined me in writing two papers. I also received some lovely correspondence following the symposium.

From Prominent Dutch contact lens specialist Esther-Simone Visser. Her father Rients Visser developed specialist scleral contact lenses.

"Dear Donald, Thank you so much for your quick and friendly answer. It is a great pleasure to read your journey to the gas permeable scleral lens. Pat Caroline has sent me images of your fitting set, I am happy to use them. I have good memories of 2008 in Las Vegas. Best wishes!"
Rients Visser

Hello Don: It was great to finally meet you - I really

> meant it when I said that I have been a fan of your work. I am glad to be able to check 'meeting Don Ezekiel at least once' off my list and hoping for more future opportunities to cross paths with you and Damon. And crossing my fingers to ask Pat to give me some of your scleral lenses so I can wow Wills Eye residents with an Ezekiel scleral lens library. Thank you!
>
> Dr Clark Chang   Wills Eye Hospital

Fort Lauderdale

I was invited to speak at a scleral lens meeting in Fort Lauderdale at the end of July. Florida was very hot and humid so Challis didn't travel with me. The featured keynote speakers were: Don Ezekiel OD on 'Scleral Lenses are Booming, But Can We Do Better?'; and Ken Pullum on 'Discoveries of the Decade'.

My papers were well received and I was often praised as being the one who made this meeting possible.

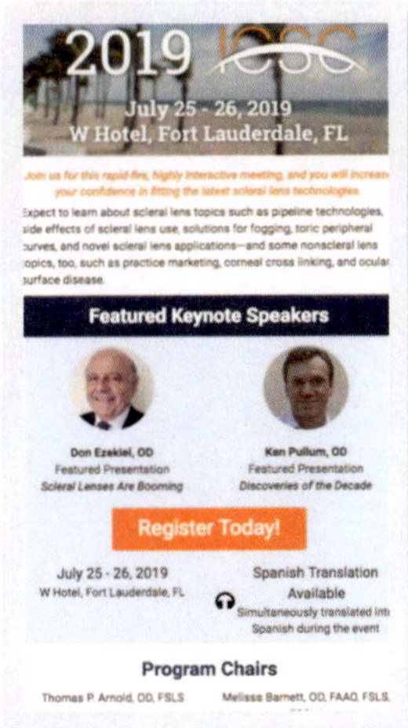

My talk described how fenestration avoided the problems caused by a sealed lens. I also presented a paper titled 'How the Gas Scleral Lens Came About'.

While I was in Fort Lauderdale, I was able to attend the world championship rowing regatta in Sarasota, Florida. Olivia had been selected in the under-23 Australian rowing team as stroke of the coxless fours, and Sasha would be there. I was able to fly to Sarasota to be there for the finals. Paul and his family flew down from New York.

They stayed at the Ritz Carlton, and Paul booked a room there for Sasha. I bunked in with her. Saturday afternoon we spent in the lagoon pool with the family. Zahara and Zed are lovely; they loved the water and Zed is a real little boy - he loved the bulldozer I bought for him! Olivia's race was early in the morning; she came third in the under 23-B. It was a good race and she was happy. It was very hot and humid. We went to a mall that was close by to recover and have lunch with Sasha and the family.

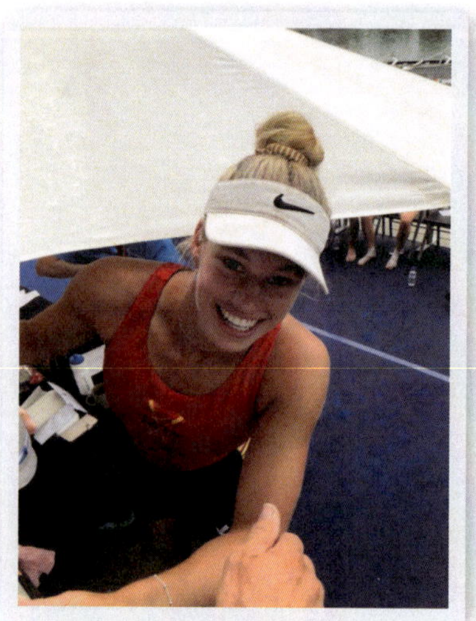
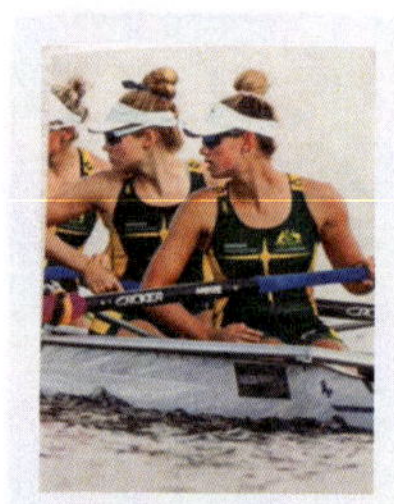

Olivia, stroke of the coxless four at the World Rowing Championships, Sarasota 2019.

Rome: ISSCL

I was invited to speak at the International Summit of Specialty Contact Lenses held in Rome in November 2019. The summit was organised by Italian-based optometrist Dr Daddi Fadel and US optometrist Dr Mindy Toabe.

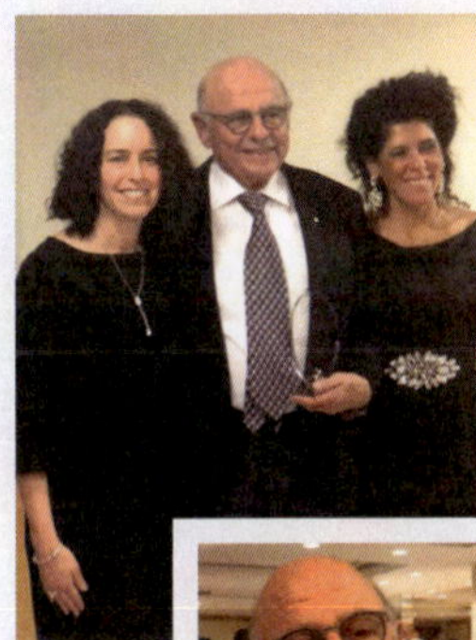

Mindy Toabe and Daddi Fadel.

Challis joined me. I read the two papers: 'The Case for Fenestrating a Scleral Lens', and 'How the Gas Permeable Scleral Lens Evolved', along with an obituary for Perry Rosenthal. All were well received. At the meeting dinner I was presented with a standing ovation, a plaque for my involvement in GP scleral lenses. It was very nice, but I was not prepared and did not speak well! There is a lot I would have liked to say and should have said. I think this will be my last meeting.

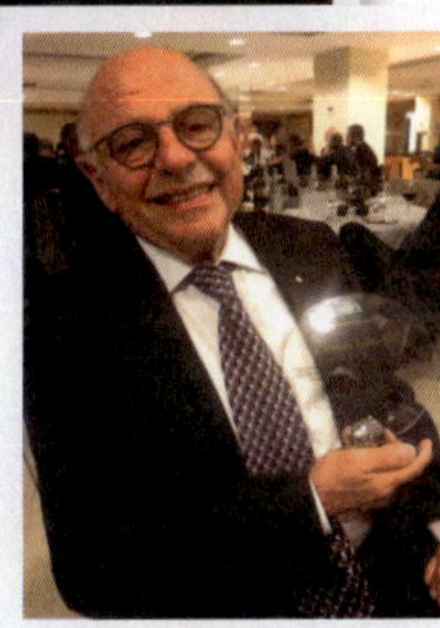

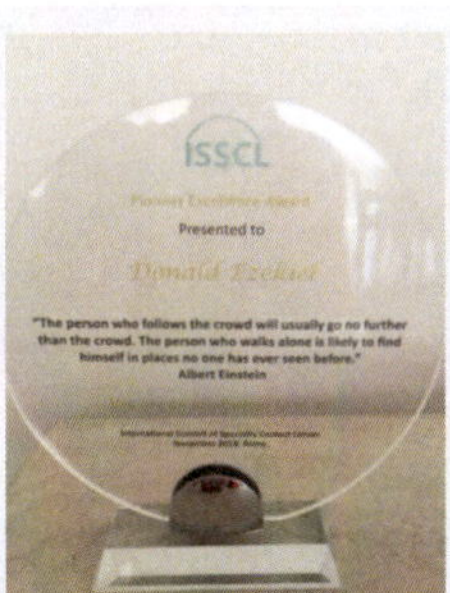

These are some emails I received from delegates at the meeting:

```
Dear Donald

You are best person I ever meet.
Thank you for sharing your
experience. Will come back to
you after seeing your document.
Thanks a lot!

Marco. (Italian Optometrist)
```

Hi Don!

It was an honour and pleasure to meet you at the AILeS meeting in Rome. Thank you for sharing this video with me... I am speechless! I cannot believe that you were fitting scleral lenses in 1983 in gas permeable material. You are truly an idol for me and someone I admire immensely. Thank you for sharing all of your valuable experience and knowledge with us. I feel truly honoured to have met you and hope to see you again in the very near future. Thank you again for all you do for our beautiful specialty and profession. Please keep in touch! Attached is a little picture of us talking.

Elise Kramer.

Dear Donald,

I would like to extend my heartfelt thanks for your participation as a speaker to AILeS Congress. It is such an honour for me and AILeS having you in the program.

The feedback from this conference was extremely positive. All responses were enthusiastic about the content and the overall quality of the conference, and we had great feedback on your presentation which fascinated all the attendees, I am really grateful for the time and effort you took to share your pioneer experiences with the attendees. I am sure that this would not have been as strong a conference without your contribution. Thank you for joining us in this "adventure". Please extend my greetings to Challis, I am deeply grateful for her effort! it was so wonderful having you both here in Rome! I hope you had a good way back home!

Warmest wishes, Daddi Faddel.'

Daddi Fadel and I co-authored two papers: 'Fenestrated Scleral Lenses. Back to the Origins Review of Their Benefits and Fitting Techniques', (published in the review journal of the American Academy of Optometry) and 'The Evolution of a Soft Translating Bifocal Lens'.

Web links to these papers are in the Appendix.

Daddi Fadel also wrote a book titled *Scleral Lens Issues and Complications* and asked me to write a forward. She also mentioned me in her list of acknowledgements.

We spent four days in Rome at the lovely Singer Palace Hotel. The hotel is a small 33-bedroom boutique hotel that was originally the office of the Singer sewing machine company. It could not be faulted. Service, food staff and the hotel itself was perfect and just a short walk to the Trevi fountain. Our friends Rita and Nigel Burnet-Hodd flew over specially to spend some time with us, which was very nice.

We then flew to New York where we spent a lovely ten days with Paul and family. Zahara and Zed are lovely. Zed is especially warm and interesting. Paul is the very best father and son. He loves the children and his dog Matilda and they love him. He checked on us each day of our visit and we loved the time we spent together.

On Shabbat I went to the Kabbalah centre with Paul, Tanya, Zahara and Zed. It was cold and wet and Challis had a bad cold so she stayed at the hotel. At the Kabbalah I had a call-up. Paul had donated a new Safer Torah to the Kabbalah centre and the service used the Torah. It is a large, very beautiful Torah. Such a mitzvah for me that the service used the Torah.

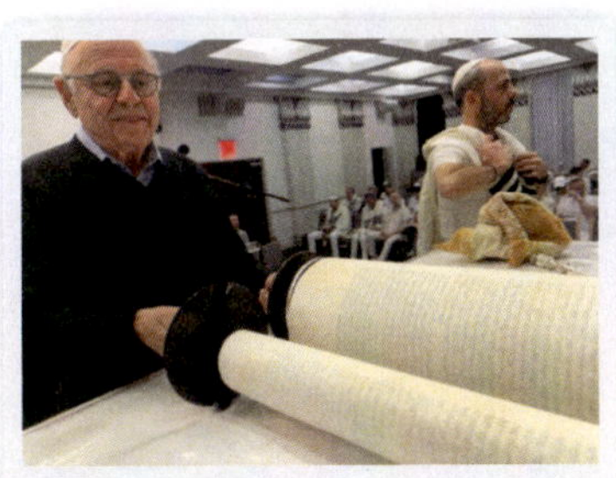

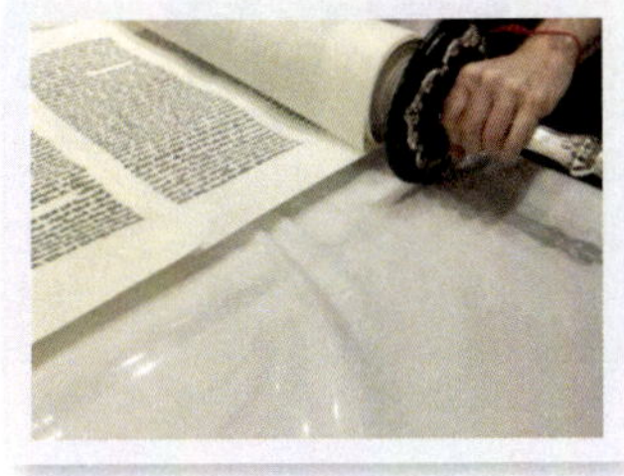

Noosa ICCLC

The following was published in *Optometry Journal:*

> The 17th conference of the ICCLC takes place in Noosa next month, featuring a line-up of world-renowned experts from the USA, Canada, Australia and New Zealand. This includes the Queen's Birthday Honours award speaker. Don Ezekiel AM, a world authority on modern scleral lenses and the recipient of the 2019 Cornea and Contact Lens Society (CCLSA) Kenneth W. Bell Award, will deliver the award, talk, and take part in a high-powered scleral lens panel session.

The Kenneth Bell Medal is interesting, as Ken was in practice in Raffles Square, Singapore, around the corner from my father's optometry practice at 13 Battery Road. We would see Ken at the Singapore Swimming Club, where he taught me how to swim.

I spoke on how the use of a gas permeable material came to be used in scleral lenses, which led to the development of the 'modern' scleral that is now available to patients worldwide. I spoke about how the sealed lens may cause problems and how fenestration of the lens eliminated these and made the lens a safe lens to wear.

Stephen Vincent, Professor of Optometry at Queensland University, presented the medal. His speech is in the Appendix.

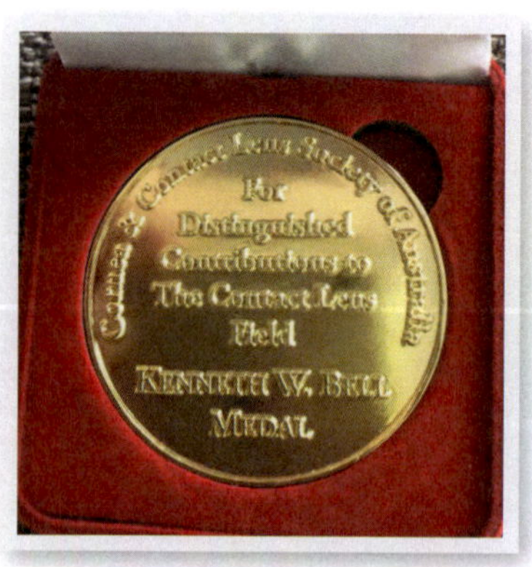

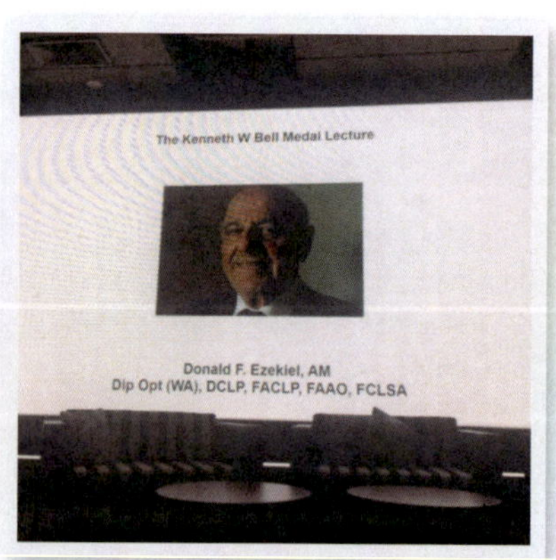

Kenneth Bell Medal.

CHAPTER TWENTY-ONE

Advanced Vision Technology

While I was in the USA, I visited Keith Parker at his laboratory, Advanced Vision Technology (AVT) in Denver. We had an agreement with Keith to make and market the custom bifocal lens.

I met with Keith and Janine Bugno, partners of AVT, and visited their laboratory. While I was there, a woman introduced herself and said she had met me when she was working with Bill Hoffman at Pangolin. Bill lived a short way from the lab so she called him and we had lunch, together with Keith's senior people. Bill looked very well and it was great to see him.

The AVT laboratory had modern technology with three DAC lathes, two with automatic loaders. The new one had a milling attachment. The lathe and mill files the technician from Gelflex had given me for the bifocal lens were in an old lathe language. Jim Marks from DAC transferred the modern lathe language. DAC was very busy and Jim did his best to get the files done for me. Really very good of him.

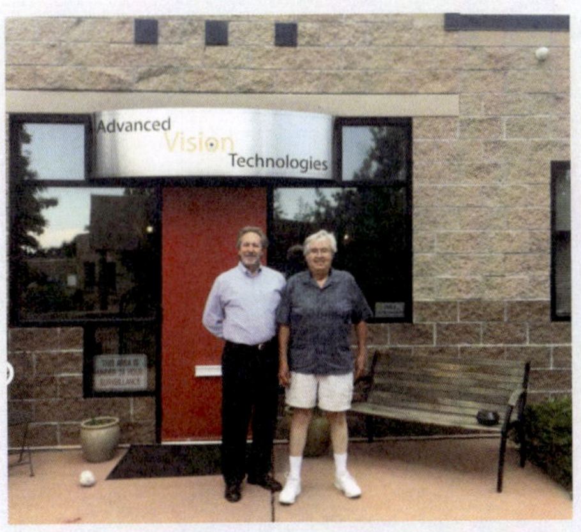

Keith Parker with Bill Hoffman.

Christine Sindt

A prominent optometrist, Christine Sindt, developed a method of taking an impression of the eye without the use of an anesthetic. Chris told me she had an idea of taking an impression and then scanning the lens to duplicate the back surface of the lens to fit the eye. Many countries do not allow optometrists to use an anesthetic but she wanted this to be available for all practitioners. She asked Ralph Stone, a prominent research doctor who I know from the ISCLS, how she could do this. As all contact lens impression systems are from dental work, he suggested she look for a retired dental scientist. Ralph later called to give Chris a name and suggested she go to a major dental meeting as he was sure to be there; she did and he was. He recommended a product that was out of patent and where she could source it.

So that was the impression method solved. Now, how to scan the impression and transfer the data to the lathe, allowing for the modification of curves as needed. For example, if the cone of a keratoconus was low and off-centre, the program would allow for the back surface to fit perfectly but allow for the front optic to be placed central to the optical area. She found the person who developed face recognition technology and he developed a program to scan the impression for her.

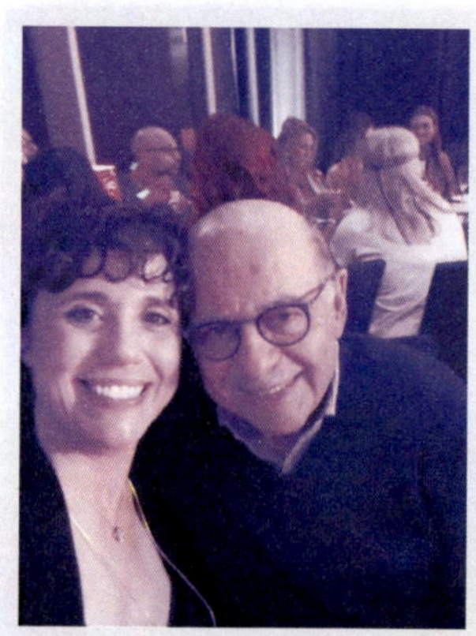

With Christine Sindt.

Keith Parker at AVT and Chris now offer this to practitioners worldwide. Very innovative. Tom Arnold had recommended AVT to me as a progressive laboratory when I was searching for a US laboratory to look at the translating bifocal lens. It was a very good choice.

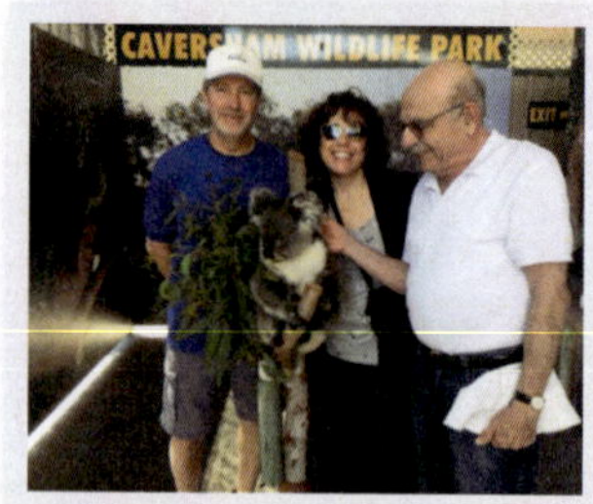

Keith Parker and Christine visiting me in Perth.

CHAPTER TWENTY-TWO

FAMILY continued

Bram's Bar Mitzvah

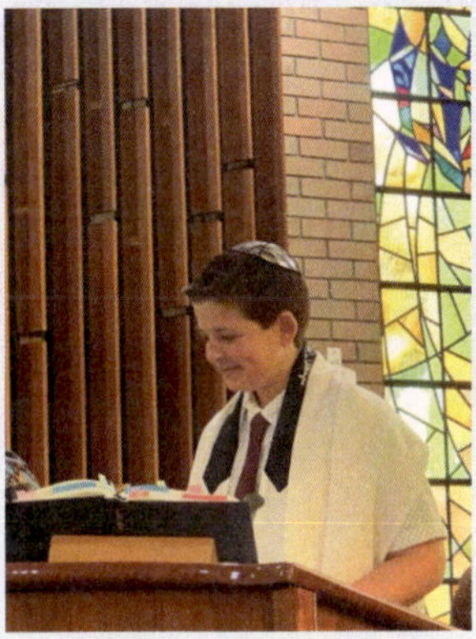

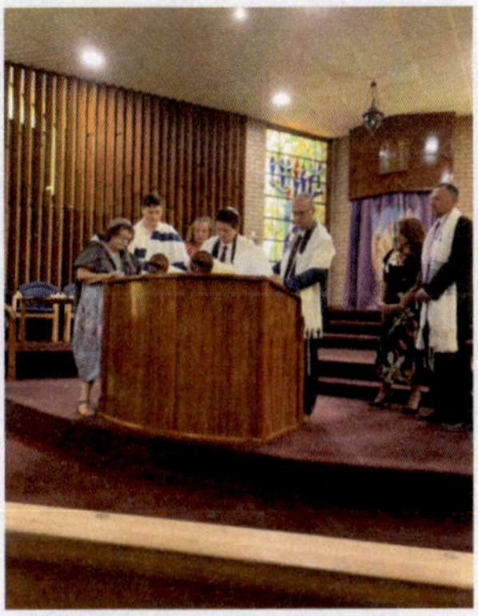

January 17th, 2020, was Bram's Bar Mitzvah. We had Shabbat dinner for him at Sasha's home, with Tania's extended family from the eastern states. The bar mitzvah was lovely. Bram took the service and spoke very well. Lunch was at the rowing club.

Singapore

The same month, Sasha went to Singapore Club Med with Max and his friend. Challis, Olivia and I flew up and met them there. We stayed at the Quincy Hotel, a five-minute walk to the Paragon Centre. Very nice, and the staff were very attentive.

While there we were invited to dinner at my cousins, Frank and Mavis Benjamin. Eddie Benjamin was there. He had had a fall and broken his leg, and was in a wheelchair. He looked old and when we left he said to me that it would be the last time we'd see him. Ten months later, in October, he passed away.

We were fortunate to have travelled when we did, as the Covid virus struck soon after we returned from Singapore and the world shut down. We all went into lockdown. Sasha brought us food and we only went out to medical appointments. Paul and his family moved to their holiday home in the Hamptons, where at least it was roomy and safe.

In July it was Challis's 80th birthday. Paul and the US family had planned to be here for her milestone, but the virus changed everything. Sasha, Olivia, Max, Tania, Romy, Bram and I went to a restaurant in the Old Treasury Buildings for dinner, which was lovely.

Selling the Apartment

We decided to sell our apartment at The Moorings. It was time to downsize, as the apartment was too far from shops and we felt isolated.

The Moorings listing was given to two prominent agents for three months exclusively, but nothing eventuated. A third agency did the apartment up very tastefully and made a wonderful brochure. The unit was sold in three weeks. The purchaser was an ex-pat living in Vancouver and didn't intend to return for five years, so we could stay in the unit until we found a suitable home to move to.

We thought we might move to a retirement village like St Louis estate, where care is available, but we wanted a three-bedroom apartment and there weren't any available. We looked at a development of new apartments being constructed around Claremont football oval, and signed on for a three-bedroom apartment at the Lucent development. It is very much smaller than The Moorings, but close to Sasha and the shops.

We moved to our new apartment at Lucent in March 2021. It is very nice. Sasha is a few minutes away, as are the shops. The folk we have met are nice and the communal lounge has been done tastefully. Every two weeks several of the ladies organise a pizza or soup night or other get together, and as we directly overlook the football oval we enjoy watching the games. A bouncing castle and food vans make it a carnival atmosphere on the weekends.

In December 2022 Paul, Tania, Zahara and Zed visited us for a couple of weeks. On the first night of Hanukah we had all the family for dinner at the Lucent residents' lounge.

CHAPTER TWENTY-THREE

THE BIFOCAL PROJECT: UPDATE

I retained all patents on the bifocal lens when the lab was sold, but was coming to the realisation that the lens may not be on the market in my lifetime.

Keith Parker at AVT was moving very slowly. Covid reduced staff time and his DAC lathes were playing up, with spare parts difficult to get.

A Chinese woman, Richel, contacted me. Her Chinese venture fund had purchased a contact lens lab in Israel. She wanted to open another one in China and was interested in the bifocal lens, both as a custom and as a disposable lens. I gave her the name of CL Tech, a UK engineering firm with an office in Singapore. They supply fully automated turnkey cast moulding and specialise in the contact lens industry. We spoke to Gordon Maccabee from CL Tech and signed a confidentiality agreement on our bifocal lens technology. He told us that a soft bifocal lens was the holy grail of contact lenses.

CL Tech use Optiform lathes, which they say are sturdier than DAC's lathes. They cut their inserts in an alloy that never needs replacing. I copied the lathe data to Gordon, who was based in Singapore. The building of the manufacturing lines happened in Southampton so Gordon sent the data there. He did a presentation to Richel of the turnkey manufacturing line he offered, and followed up with a detailed costing to make twenty or thirty 30 million lenses a year.

Gordon told Richel that the milling did not achieve a polish-free surface, but they had an idea using a system used in making the Space Lab that mills a similar hard material. He is confident this will provide a polish-free perfect truncation.

Richel wanted to know who the best people were to talk to, in order to gauge the market for the lens. I gave her the contacts for Pat Caroline, Craig Norman and Ed Bennett. I never heard back from her, so I sent her one more email saying I assumed she was not interested in pursuing the project. She eventually responded, advising us she wanted sole access to patents and design, and a royalty of 5% of sales. She also wanted lenses to evaluate, but I had given all the lenses we moulded to J&J. Gordon offered her to cast mould lenses for US$30,00, which she declined.

So I agreed to pay and Gordon refined the lens design to achieve comfort. They were very professional and much better than the ones we made. Gordon also suggested we get lenses made by a lab using his equipment to test the market before looking at making our own lenses. I tried the first lenses made and could not feel them in my eye. The UK technicians insisted that there be a blend curve between the two optics, which I wasn't happy with as this may negate the 'No Jump Optics' feature that makes the optics work so well. Further modifications were made and the drawings looked promising.

CL Tech made lenses in six powers for me to send to doctors to evaluate. Exciting times!

The lenses received from CL Tech were great. Lenses were sent to practitioners worldwide asking them to evaluate and compare them to other soft bifocal lenses now available.

One prominent US doctor replied:

> Hi Don,
>
> I was able to try the lens on a patient last week. Overall, she really liked the lens. I have to say that I am very impressed with the unique design.
>
> Best, Ashley Tucker.

I went to John Pallasis's practice and he videoed the lenses on his dispenser. John became excited - bifocal vision was 20/20 and near vision N5 with comfort.

> R +3.00 add 2.00
> L +2.00 add 2.00
> Both initially rotated vertically 90 degrees. When aligned the truncation stayed aligned with the bottom lid.
>
> With over refraction of R -0.50 L -0.25 to account for the patient's Rx
> Got 6/6 distance N6 near
> R 6/7.6 L 6/6 the patient has 0.50 cyl so good results
> Hope this helps

At the time of writing this, the bifocal project is still a work in progress. The blister-packed lenses CL Tech made were okay, but the yield was poor. The key feature for lens comfort is the truncation area. Milling the truncation, as we did at Gelflex, did not provide the required quality result for CL Tech so they used an Electro Discharge Machine to make the truncation, with varying results. I have since discovered that the electrodes differ after each process, resulting in truncations not being identical or repeatable in the tolerances needed.

I feel there must be a way to make a precise truncation that is CNC repeatable. Maybe a laser could do it?

As the CL Tech work is done in Southampton, I googled for a laser company in the UK. After checking a number of companies that offer laser cutting of metals I came across a company that could do small jobs. Their laser machine requires a special computer program for their CNC machine to recognise its computer language. CL Tech purchased the program and the truncation design with the programme sent to them. Their feedback was positive, advising their tolerances for the process was from 5 to 10 microns in all axis. I am hopeful that this will result in perfect cast moulded translating bifocal lenses with optimum yields.

I am now more hopeful that the disposable Triton lens may be a reality in my lifetime.

CHAPTER TWENTY-FOUR
REFLECTIONS OF AN INTERESTING LIFE

Now, at 87 years of age and in the twilight of my life, I have been reminiscing over my journey, and the people and events that shaped it.

I was fortunate to have taken my father's offer of a party or a trip to Singapore to see the family for my twenty-first birthday. That's when fate took me on a journey where I met Challis, who has been a wonderful wife and companion for over sixty years. Marrying Challis was one of the best decisions I ever made. She is a lovely girl and the very best wife I could have wished for. She always put up with me and my crazy dreams and ideas and fully supported them.

I regret not understanding more when my father showed early stages of mental problems, after he physically attacked me. Unfortunately I was not strong enough to appreciate that this was something he could not help. Had I realised, I could have supported him in his later years with his illness.

My father had unfortunate experiences with partners and advised me to never have a partner. He was right. My first partner was my father. That did not work out well, and we became estranged.

I then partnered with my son Damon, which also did not work out. We worked hard and tried to make it easy for him, protecting him from potential future problems with the Outram Street property, promoting him and including him as co-author of papers that he didn't contribute to. Unfortunately, it all blew up to our disadvantage. He told me he wanted the practice that I had started from scratch or he would leave. I should have told him to leave. The very profitable practice was not only keeping the lab viable, but it also meant the practice didn't have to pay tax. Damon was not happy with the profits going to the lab; he couldn't see the long-term benefit.

So he got the practice. I should have listened to Challis and not given it to him. Once the regular cash flow was lost, our financial position became very difficult and the relationship with our son became strained. Challis and I were both very hurt when Damon became estranged, and remain so.

We are fortunate to have Paul and Sasha in our lives. Paul is a good and caring son who keeps in touch with us most days. Sasha is a wonderful daughter and her children Olivia and Max are lovely and we see them often. Tania and Romy and Bram are also lovely and we feel fortunate to also have contact with them.

One of my main shortcomings has been that I was not a good businessperson. I trusted people - often the wrong people. I was always searching for people who could provide technical knowledge in contact lens manufacturing, as I had learned the manufacturing process by learning about the technology myself. Unfortunately, everyone I recruited had a personal problem that they brought with them and didn't provide any meaningful technology or effective management for the lab.

When I needed cash input for the laboratory, David Masel became a partner and CEO in the laboratory. When we were later looking for an investor in the lab, he 'arranged' for a group to buy the lab, in which he is a now partner. I got badly screwed - again.

St George Bank went from being supportive to not wanting our account. Without the debt and interest payments, and with the input of cash I was looking for, the cast moulding soft bifocal lens lab would not just have been viable, it would have been extremely profitable. I should have taken over the search for a cash infusion and spoken to other banks or groups. When we won the state and national Small Business Awards I had the opportunity to speak with several high-end companies who left me their business cards. I didn't contact any of them, as I felt I could do this on my own. I should have, as they would have contributed money (we were borrowing money at 24% interest) as well as management expertise. A percentage of something would have been better that 100% of nothing!

The market for a soft bifocal lens that provides clear vision without compromise has still never been met. The Triton soft translating bifocal lens satisfies these requirements, and I am hopeful that the lens will be available to patients - preferably in my lifetime! So, despite having just turned 87, retirement is not an option. Not just yet, anyway!

I have been very fortunate to meet so many wonderful people working in the contact lens industry around the world. They have inspired and stimulated my work.

Honorary Doctorate

In 2023, at the age of 87, I was honoured to have been awarded an Honorary Doctorate of the University of Western Australia. Receiving this award was an occasion of great personal and professional pride for me. Paul, Zahara and Zed attended the ceremony. We also invited Francis and Malcolm Steinberg, Ann and Stephen Lemonis, Barry Silbert, and Sasha and Damon's families.

The deputy chancellor presented the doctorate award.

> "You have been awarded an Honorary Doctorate of the University of Western Australia in recognition of your contribution to the private sector and the community through your work in optometry. You are an alumnus of which the University can be proud."

The award ceremony was very nice, and my valedictory speech was well received. The full version is in the Appendix.

Of all the awards I have been fortunate to receive, receiving the honorary doctorate with all my immediate family and friends present is the one that means the most to me.

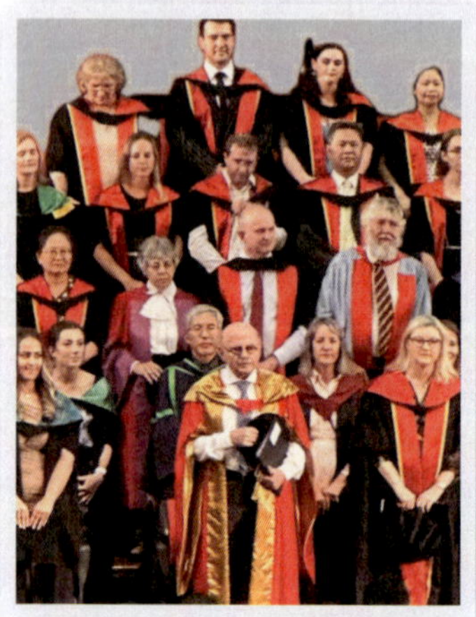

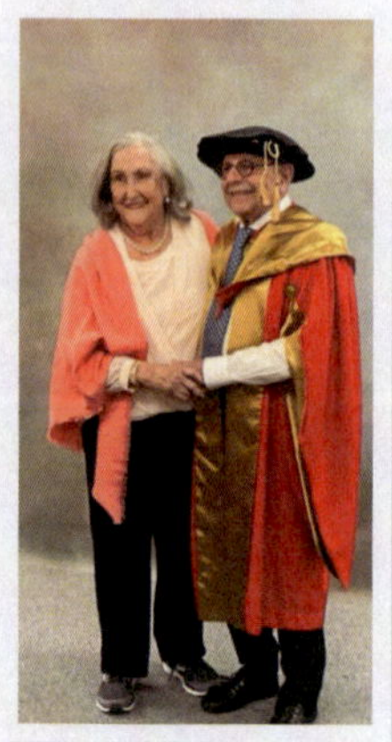

Doctorate presentation.

With Challis.

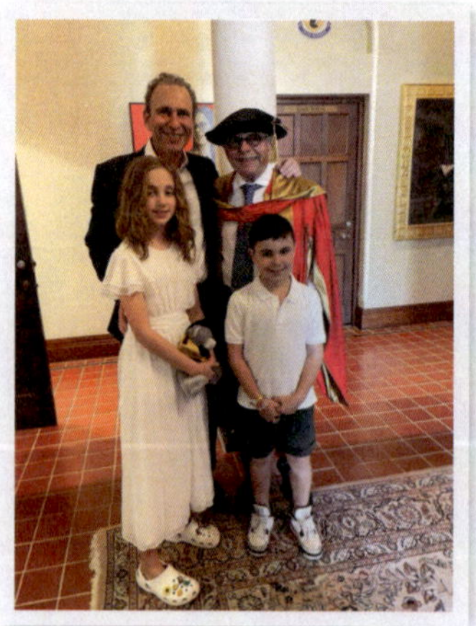

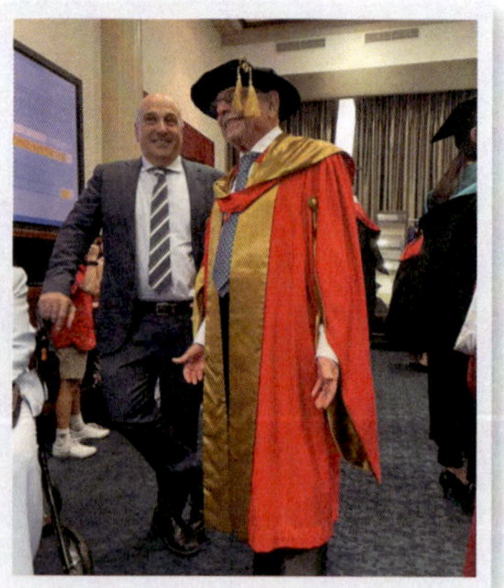

With Paul, Zahara and Zed.

Close friend Stephen Lemonis.

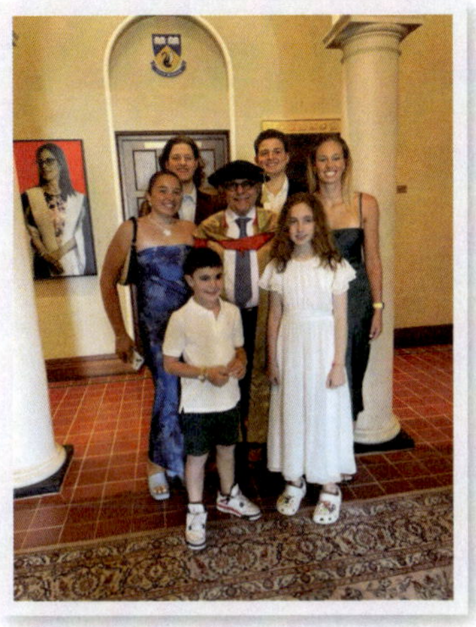

With all our grandchildren.

Our sages said, "You must leave the world in a better place than you found it."
In my own small way, maybe I have.

ACKNOWLEDGEMENTS

I wish to acknowledge all the wonderful contact lens practitioners, in Australia and around the world, who have supported me over the years. Special thanks to Patrick Caroline for his ongoing encouragement to pursue my ideas, and to John Pallasis, who undertook the evaluation of developing lenses for me.

To the suppliers of lens machinery and technology, my sincere thanks.

Many thanks to my editor Ingrid Waltham, without whose wonderful work this memoir would not have happened, and to designer Hugh Faulkner at Flametree Creative, for all his extra help and support making the book look as good as it does.

And to my ever-supportive wife Challis and family, for your understanding and unwavering support throughout all my trials and endeavours - thank you.

ABOUT THE AUTHOR

Donald Ezekiel is a world-renowned optometrist and innovator in the design and manufacture of contact lenses.

After graduating from the University of Western Australia in 1957, Don worked in the family practice in Perth before leaving for the UK to gain clinical experience. In 1963 he completed postgraduate studies in London, obtaining the Diploma in Contact Lens Practice and Fellowship of the Association of Contact Lens Practitioners. While in London Don worked alongside Josef Dallos, who trained him in the art of scleral lens manufacturing and fitting using glass.

After returning to Perth in 1970 Don established his own specialty contact lens practice and soon afterwards established Gelflex Laboratories for the research, development and manufacture of rigid and soft lenses. He did this for forty years, regularly breaking new ground within the industry and being recognised and awarded by his peers along the way. Don's many innovations included the use of rigid gas permeable materials for scleral lenses and developing what was reputedly the world's first foldable intraocular lens made from a hydrogel material. He has also worked on the development of a soft translating bifocal contact lens.

Don retired in 2012 but remains a keen and active participant in the contact lens world. He lives with his wife Challis in Claremont, a riverside suburb of Perth, Western Australia.

Career highlights:

1997: Made a Member of the Order of Australia (AM) in recognition of service to the optometry profession and to the development of the scleral contact lens.

2005: Herschel Medal, International Society of Contact Lens Specialists.

2012: Life membership, International Society of Contact Lens Specialists.

2019: The Kenneth W Bell Medal from the Australian and New Zealand Contact Lens Society, for a distinguished contribution to the field of cornea and contact lenses.

2023: Honorary Doctorate, University of Western Australia.

PEER PRAISE

"One of the greatest gifts from a professional peer is when they share their acquired knowledge, their personal experiences and the enthusiasm of their success.

"In every way this epitomises Dr Don Ezekiel, one of the great contact lens pioneers, who has so willingly, and without concern shared his wealth of knowledge with me since we first met over the twenty-five years ago. Within minutes of first meeting him in his Perth optometry practice, he was drawing diagrams to demonstrate to me how an RGP bifocal lens translates.

"This was the beginning of my own personal professional transformation as a pediatric optometrist with a postgraduate degree in orthoptics and

binocular vision, to developing a career engulfed in pediatric contact lens practice. Since then I have fitted hundreds of pediatric and adult patients with complicated RGP and scleral lens solutions, preserving their vision, all with the guidance and advice of Don at the other end. He was always there, ready and willing to help with his extensive wealth of ideas and solutions.

"Don's never-ending quest for finding and fitting the best lens for a difficult ocular problem and providing the best possible visual solution is described in this memoir. The way he overcame so many personal and professional hardships exemplifies his drive to show the world what was possible. Along the way he changed the world, producing the first gas permeable scleral lenses, paving the way for the modern scleral lenses used today.

"Don's personal journey, accompanied by his family and friends, is so interestingly portrayed in this book. The many successes and occasional failures moulded his excellent character on his way to great success. To the advantage of us all, he never gave up, enabling all professionals today to benefit from his past experience and contribution to the science.

"Dr Donald Ezekiel is definitely among the greats, and will always be remembered for his contribution to contact lenses worldwide. The privilege of having made his acquaintance and becoming a colleague and a friend is most certainly all mine."

Ivan Hare, Dip. Optom., F.O.A. (SA), D.O.B.V.(SA), M.B. C. O.(UK)
Israel Meir Hospital, Kfar Sava, Israel

***

"It is not hyperbole to state that, in many ways, Dr. Donald Ezekiel is the father of the modern contact lens. His fascinating story truly bridges the Old World with the new, and incorporates not only the technological advances that have resulted in the multitude of lens designs that we enjoy today, but the social and cultural changes that occurred along the way. Dr. Ezekiel enumerates his family's struggle through World War II, his parents relocation to Singapore, and then the family's move to Western Australia, where Don built his remarkable career.

"Ever indefatigable, Dr. Ezekiel is still innovating and creating new designs to meet the needs of patients whatever they may be. His journey is truly nonpareil and sure to hold the reader's attention."

Thomas P. Arnold, OD, FSLS
Loveland, Colorado, USA

***

"Donald Ezekiel's memoir is a captivating journey through the life of an optometry trailblazer who overcame humble beginnings to revolutionise the field with a flair for innovation, introducing game-changing creations like gas permeable scleral lenses.

"Through his compelling narrative, Ezekiel's enduring legacy as a visionary in the field comes to life. It is a fascinating and inspiring read."

Dr. Elise Kramer, OD

Fellow of the American Academy of Optometry, the Scleral Lens Education Society, and the BCLA

Public Education Chair, Scleral Lens Education Society (SLS)

Delegate of International Relations, AILeS

Former resident at the Miami VAMC and Bascom Palmer Eye Institute 2012-13

APPENDIX 1

IDA MANN/DALLOS LETTER

CONTACT LENSES AND DR. JOSEF DALLOS.

Contact lenses are not new. In 14 years we shall be celebrating their centenary, for it was in 1887 that Professor Saemisch suggested to Müller, a glass eye manufacturer, of Wiesbaden, that he could blow a glass shell for a patient whose eyelids had been partly lost through disease and who could not close his eye. This patient wore his lens for 21 years with no damage to his cornea and with good tolerance. This showed that the idea was a sound one and research was well under way by 1892 when the firm of Zeiss began to produce mathematically accurate haptic lenses in all powers. At the same time the Japanese were experimenting with blown glass lenses and achieving some success but at the expense of a most time-consuming process. These lenses had a thin corneal portion and thick hollow outer scleral rim (rather like a little sausage) running round the periphery. They were large and their optical properties were far from perfect. Very many had to be blown for each patient before one, both comfortable and optically acceptable was produced. They were soon superceded by the various European types.

It is to Josef Dallos that we owe much. He made it possible to obtain an accurate and a comfortable fit combined with a perfect optical portion. Dallos, a Hungarian of Jewish extraction, was working on the contact lens problem in Budapest. He concentrated on research on moulded glass lenses. The idea of moulded lenses began in 1888 when Fick experimented with various moulding materials. Little success was achieved until Csapody, in 1929, had the idea of using Dentacoll, a soft substance employed by dentists for taking casts of the mouth. Dallos investigated this and developed the method of taking casts of eyes using a similar substance, Negocoll.

Before this, the firm of Zeiss were perfecting their glass lenses. I first saw a patient wearing these with

-2-

comfort at the Amsterdam meeting of the International Ophthalmological Congress in the early 1920's but they **proved** far from universally applicable.

The next advance came in 1938 when Obrig introduced the plastic lens. By this time Dallos was in some jeopardy from the political troubles in Hungary which were beginning at that time.

In 1937 three English ophthalmologists, Mr. Williamson-Noble, Mr. Rugg Gunn and myself decided to put ourselves under Dallos for instruction in the method of fitting from a mould and subsequent hand grinding of the glass shell to obtain a comfortable fit. We went to Budapest and learned the technique but soon realised the amount of practice required and the time-consuming nature of the work which would have left us, as Dallos had found, no time for the pursuit of general ophthalmology.

In 1938 the menace of Hitler made it obvious that if Dallos' pioneer and very successful work was to continue he must leave Hungary. The firm of Hamblin, Dispensing Opticians, of Wigmore Street, had offered to set up a contact lens centre in Cavendish Square, attached to their Wigmore Street premises, if we could persuade Dallos to come to England.

I went to Budapest again in 1938 to argue with Dallos over the proposition. It was a tricky psychological situation. Dallos was torn between his desire as an Hungarian to remain in his laboratory and his wish to continue his work in peace in England, unassailed by political menace. I felt that if Dallos' genius were lost to England and the world the development of contact lenses would be delayed indefinitely.

I well remember driving in a taxi with Dallos round and round Budapest, arguing and persuading in an emotional storm of protestation, entreaty, dismay, regret and finally tears, as the necessity for becoming a refugee slowly dawned

-3-

on him. I won my point and he was soon established in London in the first Contact Lens Centre in England under the supervision of Williamson-Noble, Rugg Gunn and myself as a sort of committee of management.

Many improvements resulted. The fenestrated lens, the plastic lens and refinements in fitting. Dallos set the scene for contact lens work in England. To his dedicated attitude to the work and his single-mindedness over the problems we owe the foundation of all the contact lens centres of today, but his somewhat difficult character has, I feel, prevented him from attaining full recognition of his genius. He was always loth to publish or to attend and speak at meetings. He found it difficult to pass on his knowledge, though many have succeeded in learning from him. One of his pupils, Mr. Philip J. Beilby, came to Western Australia after the war and amazed us by restoring to full employment 20 patients whose corneal disabilities had put them on Invalid Pensions.

Today, of course, in England all the large eye hospitals have departments: contact lens fitters abound, successful wearers of cosmetic, occupational and medical lenses are numbered in thousands and ideas and techniques continue to proliferate in England, Australia and America. Meanwhile, Dallos, shy as ever, continues his work in a small laboratory in London, now divorced from Hamblin's. One group of his patients at least will never forget him - the 84 victims of delayed mustard gas keratitis (from the first World War) whom he restored to sight and comfort around 1940-44.

And we three ophthalmologists will never regret that we persuaded him to leave Hungary for England and thus to lay the foundation of our present contact lens work.

Ida Mann.

---oOo--- Aug. 1973.

APPENDIX 2

Article written by Nathan Efron for *Clinical and Experimental Optometry*, 2014.

Donald Ezekiel AM: passionate and innovative contact lens practitioner and manufacturer.

Donald Ezekiel (known to all as 'Don') was born in Singapore on September 12, 1936, to a German mother and Iraqi father. His parents were Jewish refugees, who met in Batavia, married and alternately lived in Batavia and Singapore. The family established their primary residence in Singapore after Don's older brother Eric (later to become a haematologist) was born in 1934. The Ezekiel family was forced to flee in 1941 when the Japanese bombed Singapore and were fortunate to obtain passage on a hospital ship to Perth. They returned to Singapore after the war but left again on their own accord in 1951 due to race riots. The Ezekiels sold up everything in Singapore and decided to settle in Perth.

Don's father was a prominent optometrist who had practices in Batavia and Singapore and when he arrived in Australia established a small practice in Perth. Don followed in his father's footsteps, graduating with a Diploma in Optometry from the Optometry Board of Western Australia in 1957. He worked in the family practice of 'M. Ezekiel and Sons' in Perth before travelling to Melbourne to gain experience with the esteemed optometric establishment Coles and Garrard. Don began to develop an interest in contact lenses and in 1960 he travelled to Sydney to be taught scleral lens fitting by Lloyd Hewett.

➢ Seeking Further Contact Lens Knowledge

Don was aware that great leaps forward in the contact lens field were taking place in the UK. So in 1963, only four days after marrying Challis, Don and his new wife travelled to London, where Don enthusiastically set about gaining a wide variety of clinical experiences. In a wise strategic move, he sought to establish credibility in the field and embarked upon postgraduate studies, obtaining his Diploma in Contact Lens Practice and Fellowship of the Association of Contact Lens Practitioners. He recalls gaining invaluable experience, while attending a contact lens course at City University conducted by Robert Fletcher, head of optometry and later professor.

Now Don has a charming demeanour, infectious smile and hearty laugh, and he seems to have used these traits to great effect by endearing himself to various luminaries in the field. Before going to London, Don held a position as honorary optometrist at the Royal Perth Hospital. He used that connection to obtain an introduction to Frederick Ridley, who was head of Moorfields Eye Hospital. Ridley introduced Don to his registrar, Montague ('Monty') Ruben, who was later to become head of the renowned contact lens clinic at Moorfields. Ruben warmed to Don and allowed him to sit in on the hospital's contact lens clinics. Don also met Norman Bier at Moorfields and the two became good friends. Bier was an English optometrist and author of one of the earliest contact lens textbooks.

Don also needed to earn a living, so he applied for a position at Hamblin's famous New Cavendish Street practice. The staff there advised Don that the head of the contact lens clinic—the legendary Josef Dallos —was a difficult man to work with and rarely employed people, preferring to work alone. Undeterred, Don gained an interview and was offered a job. He found Dallos to be a lovely, warm man and a great teacher; however, working for Dallos posed considerable technical challenges. Although there was a growing trend for scleral lenses to be fabricated from polymethyl methacrylate (PMMA), Dallos preferred to work with glass. Don once told me the story of when he had spent countless hours carefully grinding a glass scleral lens into shape for a patient and noticed during the fitting visit that there was still slightly too much bearing upon a small region of the sclera. He proceeded to carefully grind just a little more off the lens edge, when all of a sudden the lens totally shattered into tiny fragments, meaning that he had to start all over again. This sort of accident occurred frequently, making glass lens manufacture heartbreaking work.

Dallos taught Don a great deal but two pieces of advice in particular were to have a profound effect on Don's future career. First, never trust the quality and dimensions of lenses made for you by laboratories; if you really care for your patients, you should make your own lenses. Second, undertake research to test your ideas.

During Don's initial interview with Dallos, he was asked if he knew the renowned British ophthalmologist, Professor Dame Ida Mann, who had migrated to Perth in the early 1950s. Don replied that not only did he know her, but Dame Ida was living in the Perth suburb of Dalkeith, where Don also lived. When Don returned to Perth, he called Dame Ida to pass on Dallos's good wishes, and spent many interesting hours speaking with her.

On one occasion, Don told Dame Ida that the annual meeting of the Contact Lens Society of Australia was to be held in Perth and that he was presenting a paper. She asked when and where and to his surprise, she attended. This was at a time when ophthalmologists declined to have anything to do with optometry. Don fondly recalls acknowledging her presence before presenting his paper. Dame Ida died in 1983 and in 2012, Don was invited to London to unveil an English Heritage Blue Plaque identifying Dame Ida's former place of residence.

After their initial stay in London, Don and Challis travelled around Europe and Don took the opportunity to engage in further networking, meeting up with well-known European practitioners, including Pierre Rocher.

Don returned to Perth and in 1970 established his own practice specialising in contact lenses. The following year he travelled back to London to purchase the machinery required to make his own lenses. By this time, soft contact lenses had arrived on the scene, so Don decided to learn how to fabricate these lenses too. In London, he met George Nissel, a prominent manufacturer of machinery that could be used to fabricate both rigid and soft lenses. He also met up with Philip Cordrey and David Clulow, who owned Contact Lens Manufacturing, which produced Sauflon contact lenses and solutions. Cordrey and Clulow showed Don how to manufacture high water contact lenses and contact lens solutions.

➢ Ezekiel, The Contact Lens Manufacturer

After returning from his second trip to London in 1971, Don started to manufacture contact lenses for his patients. The laboratory was initially called Western Australian Contact Lens Manufacturing, but this was later changed to Gelflex Laboratories. This company also represented Sauflon in Australia.

Soon after the laboratory was established, Gelflex and three other Australian companies received a high court writ from the New York-based National Patent Development Corporation, claiming that these companies had infringed a patent owned by NPDC describing the manufacture of a soft lens in a rigid form and then hydrating the rigid form to create a soft lens, which was the process Don was using at Gelflex Laboratories. Two of the companies that received the writ were lens importers and immediately complied by ceasing operation. The third company that received the writ was Sydney-based Corneal Lens Corporation, owned by optometrist Penhryn Thomas. Corneal Lens Corporation allowed itself to be acquired by Hydron—a company wholly owned by NPDC—which left Don to defend the writ alone. Many overseas academics and scientists forwarded documents to Don, demonstrating that there was prior knowledge to the art. Don's legal team presented this information to the high court and nothing further was heard. This was an important early lesson for Don in the murky business of patent protection and litigation and what companies would do to protect their market.

Today, Gelflex Laboratories manufactures soft and rigid lenses. The company also houses Australia's first and only cast moulding facility. Gelflex Laboratories was awarded the West Australian State and Australian National Small Business awards in 1984. The company was acquired by an investment group in 2012, at which time Don retired from contact lens manufacturing.

➢ Ezekiel, The Contact Lens Innovator

As a skilled practitioner with his own manufacturing laboratory, Don has always been in a unique position to innovate, fabricate lenses and conduct experiments, just as Dallos advised. It is not possible to detail all of Don's inventions, so by way of example I shall highlight three developments of particular interest.

Don presented a paper at the 1983 meeting of the British Contact Lens Association in Harrogate, UK, where he described fitting forty-three patients with scleral lenses manufactured from rigid gas permeable materials. This was the first time RGP scleral lens fitting had been described. Don suggests that this was not 'rocket science' but a normal progression, as at the time almost all rigid lenses were being fabricated from gas permeable materials, so it was logical that these materials should be used for scleral lenses. Nevertheless, it was an important development because up until this time scleral lenses had been fabricated from glass or PMMA, both of which were impermeable to oxygen. Such lenses could only be worn for four to six hours at a time before hypoxic-induced oedema made lens wear intolerable. RGP scleral lenses represented a significant advance as they allowed greater corneal oxygenation and longer wearing times. Ophthalmologist and co-founder of Polymer Technology Corporation, Perry Rosenthal, describes Don as the 'father of gas permeable scleral lenses'.

In the mid-1980s, working with Graham Barrett—then a young registrar in ophthalmology at the Royal Perth Hospital—Don developed what was reputedly the world's first foldable intraocular lens, made from a hydrogel material using techniques adapted from his contact lens manufacturing processes. The key advantage of a foldable intraocular lens is that a much smaller limbal incision is required to insert the lens into the eye. The patent for this development was licensed to Alcon laboratories.

Don has developed and patented a soft translating bifocal contact lens. All currently available soft bifocal lenses work on the principle of simultaneous distance/near correction, which is a sub-optimal optical compromise. In some respects, Don's invention is a logical extension of what happens with rigid lenses, whereby the lens translates over the cornea, so that the appropriate optical portion of the lens will be positioned in front of the pupil to effect clear near or distance vision; however, translation of the lens is affected by interaction with the lids, and lid-lens interactions are known to be a primary source of contact lens discomfort. Don Ezekiel is an innovator and lateral thinker and apparently has been able to design this lens such that it causes minimal discomfort. Although the original concept was first described 14 years ago, Don still believes that a disposable form of this lens, which can be mass-manufactured using cast moulding, will become available in the not too distant future. Only time will tell if this eventuates and the lens becomes a market success.

➢ Recognition and Honours

In 1997, Don was made a Member of the Order of Australia (AM) 'in recognition of service to the optometric profession and to the development of the scleral contact lens'.

The International Society of Contact Lens Specialists awarded the Herschel Medal to Don in 2005 and bestowed him with honorary life membership in 2012.

One of Don's key interests outside optometry is magic and he has served as President of the Western Australian Magic Society.

Don is now semi-retired and still engages in contact lens consulting. The Ezekiel optometric dynasty now extends to three generations, as Don's son Damon practices optometry in Perth.

Don has been a passionate and innovative contact lens practitioner and manufacturer and his many contributions have served to enhance the art and science of contact lens practice locally, nationally and internationally. Such is his standing in the field that Don's contributions are referred to in no less than nine pages of Tim Bowden's authoritative tome documenting the history of contact lenses. Sadly, in this modern world of mass production and global marketing of contact lenses, we are unlikely to benefit in the future from contributions of entrepreneurial individuals of the likes of Donald Ezekiel.

APPENDIX 3.

THE KENNETH BELL AWARD

Presentation Speech delivered by Professor Stephen Vincent, Queensland Institute of Optometry.

The Kenneth W Bell Medal is awarded to a CCLSA member in recognition of their distinguished contribution to the field of cornea and contact lenses. This morning it's my privilege to introduce this year's recipient, Don Ezekiel, AM. Don is a world-renowned optometrist and contact lens manufacturer, but has been described by many as an expert, innovator, inventor, lateral thinker, a passionate pioneer and, the grandfather of gas permeable scleral lenses.

Don graduated from the University of Western Australia in 1957 and began his journey with scleral lenses in 1960 with Lloyd Hewett, a Sydney-based optometrist and leader in the contact lens field. In 1963 Don completed postgraduate studies in London obtaining the Diploma in Contact Lens Practice and Fellowship of the Association of Contact Lens Practitioners. During this time abroad he also worked alongside the legendary Josef Dallos, who trained Don in the art of scleral lens manufacturing and fitting using glass.

In 1970 Don opened his own specialty contact lens practice in Perth, Western Australia and soon afterwards, on the advice from Dallos, Bier, and Ruben (the Northern hemisphere scleral pioneers), established Gelflex Laboratories for research and development and the manufacture of rigid and soft lenses for his patients, where he continued to challenge and advance our industry over the next 40 years.

In these early years of practice Don would treat and manufacture lenses for all manner of patients referred from local ophthalmologists including infant aphakes which would require Don to attend theatre and take a mould of the eye. To simplify this process, based on his previous clinical experience, Don simply calculated the most common scleral lens parameters required in such cases and manufactured standard paediatric scleral lenses in two diameters both with a back vertex power of +30 D. All aphakic babies were fitted in these particular designs, and the as the child and their eye grew, the power was simply modified by grinding down the same lens.

A series of events in the early 1980's involving Don have arguably influenced many practitioners in this very room. At the time, contact lens fitting had shifted primarily towards soft lenses, and corneal rigid lenses had evolved from PMMA to gas permeable materials. However, Don was still fitting fenestrated PMMA sclerals in numerous cases of advanced keratoconus with decentred cones, post-graft corneas, and as a protective device in cases of recalcitrant dry eye and lid deformities.

In Don's mind, the next logical step in contact lens evolution was to manufacture sclerals in gas permeable materials. Despite being met with significant resistance, for example being told that "nobody fits sclerals anymore", Don persisted. He travelled the globe and eventually secured large enough blanks in gas permeable materials from the United States to manufacture his own RGP scleral lenses. Don transitioned his existing PMMA scleral wearers across to RGP materials enhancing oxygen delivery to the cornea, improving comfort and extending wearing time. And the rest is history.

Around the same time, in the mid-80s, while working with an ophthalmology registrar at the Royal Perth Hospital, Don developed what was reputedly the world's first foldable intraocular lens, made from a hydrogel material rather than PMMA, using techniques adapted from his contact lens manufacturing processes. The key advantage of a foldable IOL was that a much smaller limbal incision was required to insert the lens. Don also developed a translating soft bifocal contact lens. The Triton lens was developed in order to improve vision for both distance and near visual tasks as an alternative to various simultaneous vision bifocal lenses.

In 1997, Don was made a Member of the Order of Australia 'in recognition of service to optometry and the development of the scleral contact lens'. He was awarded the Herschel Medal from the International Society of Contact Lens Specialists in 2005 in recognition of "outstanding original contributions to contact lens design techniques, the education of students, and the advancement of the status of contact lens practice." He was also bestowed honorary life membership by the same organisation in 2012. In 2015, Don received the Award of Excellence at The Global Specialty Lens Symposium in the United States for his enduring contributions to the contact lens industry. And today we are very pleased to announce Don as the 2019 Kenneth W Bell medallist.

APPENDIX 4.

PUBLISHED PAPERS

In 1963 I presented a paper on 'Gas Permeable Materials to Manufacture Haptic Lenses' at the annual meeting of the British Contact Lens Society in Harrogate. It was the first time a paper had been read and published on the use of GP materials for scleral lenses and resulted in my being called the 'Grandfather of the gas permeable scleral lens'. The paper was published in the *Journal of the British Contact Lens Association,* Vol. 6. No. 4

https://www.sciencedirect.com/sdfe/pdf/download/eid/1-s2.0-S0141703783800640/first-page-pdf

Daddi Fadel and I co-authored two papers: *Fenestrated Scleral Lenses. Back to the Origins Review of Their Benefits and Fitting Techniques*, (published in the review journal of the American Academy of Optometry) and *The Evolution of a Soft Translating Bifocal Lens.*

They can be found here:

https://journals.lww.com/optvissci/abstract/2020/09000/fenestrated_scleral_lenses__back_to_the_origins_.22.aspx

https://meroeye.com/news/the-evolution-of-a-soft-translating-bifocal-lens/

In 1998 I wrote a paper with Damon on the scepticism that existed around rigid gas permeable scleral lenses:

https://www.clspectrum.com/issues/1998/december/overcoming-skepticism-about-rgp-scleral-lenses/

APPENDIX 5.

AMERICAN ACADEMY OF OPTOMETRY

In 1984, I was invited by the American Optometry to make a presentation on gas permeable scleral lenses, at an AAO symposium in St Louis, Missouri.

F.A. A.O.

AMERICAN ACADEMY of OPTOMETRY

THE CORNEA AND CONTACT LENS SECTION

CHAIRMAN
MICHAEL G. HARRIS, O.D., M.S.
School of Optometry
University of California
Berkeley, California 94720
415-642-5761

SECTION EXECUTIVE COMMITTEE

IMMEDIATE PAST PRESIDENT
SHELDON WECHSLER, M. Opt., O.D.
P.O. Box 10167
Jacksonville, Florida 32207
[illegible]
VICE CHAIRMAN
RICHARD D. BRANNEN, O.D.
[illegible]
[illegible], New Hampshire [illegible]
[illegible]
SECRETARY
C.A. BAYSHORE, O.D.
[illegible]
Orlando, Florida 32804
[illegible]
PROGRAM CHAIRMAN
RODGER T. KAME, O.D.
[illegible] East First Street, Suite [illegible]
Los Angeles, California [illegible]
[illegible]
COURSES CHAIRMAN
[illegible], O.D.
[illegible] Street
Orlando, Florida [illegible]
[illegible]
DIPLOMATE AWARD CHAIRMAN
GERALD E. LOWTHER, O.D., Ph.D.
College of Optometry
Ferris State College
Big Rapids, Michigan [illegible]
[illegible]

[illegible] CHAIRMAN
STEPHEN [illegible], O.D.
[illegible]
San Francisco, California [illegible]

23 [illegible]

March 15, 1984

Donald Ezekiel, O.D.
Western Australia Contact Lens Manufacturing
43 Outram Street
West Perth, Australia 6005

Dear Doctor Ezekiel:

As a result of a recent conversation with Dr. Melvin Remba, I write to ask if you might be interested in reporting on your experience on the application and efficacy of gas permeable scleral lenses. The contact lens program of the American Academy of Optometry is to be held on Tuesday morning December 11, 1984 in St. Louis, Missouri. The symposium is entitled "Contemporary and Innovative Contact Lens Procedures".

Even though the concept of the gas permeable sclerals have been discussed in the past, I understand you have taken the initiative and implemented this concept.

The Cornea and Contact Lens Section would be honored to have you present a lecture of approximately one-half hour as part of this symposium.

I look forward to hearing from you. A reply by April 15, would be greatly appreciated.

Sincerely,

Rodger T. Kame, O.D.,F.A.A.O.
Program Chairman
RTK/ii

F.A. A.O.

AMERICAN ACADEMY of OPTOMETRY

THE CORNEA AND CONTACT LENS SECTION

24 APR 1984

April 8, 1984

Donald F. Ezekiel, O.D.
43 Outram Street
West Perth, Australia 6005

Dear Doctor Ezekiel:

It was nice to hear from you and about the optimism you hold towards gas permeable haptic lenses.

I would say that many of us here in the United States are serious about the possibilities of such lenses and "thirst" for more concrete information. A presentation by you would certainly be a welcomed addition to the Tuesday program of the Cornea and Contact Lens Section entitled "Contemporary and Innovative Contact Lens Procedures".

Insofar as expenses are concerned, I regret that the Academy does not have resources for these research papers and reports given.

May I suggest that you also submit a proposal immediately, as the deadline is sometime in April, for a Ellerbrock Continuing Education Lecture and/workshop to be given prior to the Academy Papers Meeting. Attendees are charged for these courses and you could receive a sizeable monetary compensation depending on the number of enrolled. Should you decide to submit a course proposal, it should be addressed to:

Dr. Jess Boyd Eskridge
The University of Alabama of Birmingham
The Medical Center/School of Optometry
University Station
Birmingham, Alabama 35294
Telephone (205) 934-4488

Please send a copy to:

Dr. William Lee
214 East Marks Street
Orlando, Flordia 32803

F.A. A.O.

AMERICAN ACADEMY of OPTOMETRY

THE CORNEA AND CONTACT LENS SECTION

June 7, 1984

RECEIVED 18 JUN 1984

Dr. Donald F. Ezekiel
43 Outram Street
West Perth, Australia 6005

Dear Dr. Ezekiel,

This is to confirm your participation on the Tuesday, December 11, 1984 program of the Cornea and Contact Lens Section of the American Academy of Optometry. The Section is delighted that you would be willing to give of your time and expense to advance the science of contact lens technology.

As you may know the Academy program is research oriented and we request that your presentation be submitted for publication in the Archives. For program printing purposes I would appreciate your subject title, an abstract of course content, and your name, degrees, institution, and city as you would like it to appear in the program. Please mail this information to me by July 1st.

Plan to allow five minutes for questions and answers at the conclusion of your presentation.

The tentative schedule is:

Symposium: CONTEMPORARY AND INNOVATIVE CONTACT LENS PROCEDURES

8:00 - 8:30 AM	Gas Permeable Scheral Lenses. Donald F. Ezekiel,OD,West Perth, Australia.
8:30 - 9:00	Hydrogel Alternative For Color Defective. Jay Schlanger,OD,Los Angeles, CA.
9:00 - 9:30	Use of Prosthetic and Cosmetic Lenses In Contemporary Practice. Joe Shovlin, OD, Harrisburg, PA.
9:30 -10:00	Novel GP and Gel Combination Lens. Bert Corwin,OD,Rapid City,So. Dakota.
10:00 - 10:30	Specialized Fitting of Rare Patients:"Piggyback" Lenses and Aphakic Pediatric Cases. Barry Weissman,OD,Ph.D.,Jules Stein Eye Institute,L.A.,CA.
10:30 - 11:00	Recent Studies in Keratoconus. A.E. Reynolds,OD,MD, Ph.D.,Tulsa, OK.
11:00 - 11:30	The Role of Contact Lenses In Radial·Keratotomy. Sami El Hage, OD, Ph.D., Houston, Texas.

Cordially,

Rodger T. Kame, O.D., F.A.A.O.

RTK:mf
cc: Drs. Harris & Brannen

F.A. A.O.

AMERICAN ACADEMY of OPTOMETRY

THE CORNEA AND CONTACT LENS SECTION

CHAIRMAN
MICHAEL G. HARRIS, O.D., M.S.
School of Optometry
University of California
Berkley, California 94720
415-642-5761

SECTION EXECUTIVE COMMITTEE

IMMEDIATE PAST PRESIDENT
SHELDON WECHSLER, M. Opt., O.D.
P.O. Box 10157
Jacksonville, Florida 32207
800-874-5278
VICE CHAIRMAN
RICHARD D. BRANNEN, O.D.
313 Nugget Arcade
Hanover, New Hampshire 03755
603-643-2140
SECRETARY
C.A. BAYSHORE, O.D.
2013 Countryside Cir. So.
Orlando, Florida 32804
305-423-2323
PROGRAM CHAIRMAN
RODGER T. KAME, O.D.
250 East First Street, Suite 800
Los Angeles, California 90012-3875
213-626-7419
COURSES CHAIRMAN
WM. C. LEE, O.D.
214 E. Marks Street
Orlando, Florida 32803
305-841-6220
DIPLOMATE AWARD CHAIRMAN
GERALD E. LOWTHER, O.D., Ph.D.
College of Optometry
Ferris State College
Big Rapids, Michigan 49307
616-796-0461 ext 3023

CASE REPORTS CHAIRMAN
STEPHEN LESTER, O.D.
760 Market St.
San Francisco, California 94102
415-392-2267

December 27, 1984

Donald F. Ezekiel, O.D.
43 Outram Street
West Perth 6005, Western Australia

Dear Doctor Ezekiel,

On behalf of the Cornea and Contact Lens Section of the American Academy of Optometry, I wish to thank you for your participation in the Section Symposium at our recently held meeting in Saint Louis.

Your contribution to the advancement of knowledge in our mutual area of interest is greatly appreciated. Furthermore your willingness to share your knowledge with others attests to your dedication to the advancement of the field of contact lenses and related sciences.

Sincere best wishes in the coming year. May it prove to be a most fruitful one for you.

Cordially,

Rodger T. Kame, O.D., F.A.A.O.
1984 Program Chairman

RTK:mf
cc: Drs. Poster, Brannen, Lowther

SECTION COMMITTEE

MICHAEL FRIEDBERG, O.D.
MORTON KAY, O.D.
DONALD KORB, O.D.
CLARENCE L. McEACHERN, O.D.
DONALD A. SPRINGER, O.D.
CHARLES STEWART, O.D., Ph.D.
SOL TABAK, O.D.
C. EDWARD WILLIAMS, O.D.

AND ALL PAST CHAIRMEN

APPENDIX 6.

SUCCESS STORIES

A see-through solution

When Joseph Dallos, the 'father' of the contact lens, said, "it doesn't matter what you do, you can always do it better", it was the beginning of success for optometrist Don Ezekiel.

That advice, coupled with his desire to help patients, led Ezekiel to making lenses that are putting him on the global map.

As a young optometrist in 1971, Ezekiel visited Britain which was then using ocular materials unavailable in Australia. His British colleagues gave him the connections for both the raw materials and the process, and talked him into making his own lenses in Perth.

Early lenses were made from glass and Perspex. Then came a gas permeable material which allowed the eye to 'breathe'. By this stage, around 1979, Ezekiel was manufacturing lenses at his Gelflex Laboratories in Perth. It was a logical evolution that scleral lenses be made from these breathing materials.

Ezekiel approached the manufacturer in the United States, asking for the gas permeable material to be supplied in a format big enough to make the large scleral lenses.

"I was told that it was only available in 'small buttons' for little lenses and nobody made the large scleral lenses any more. But I persisted. The Americans made the big buttons for me."

In 1983 at the British Contact Lens Society Ezekiel described his results. His lens, he said, could get oxygen to the eye. But his paper was disregarded, even though the Britons were looking for a way to get oxygen to the eyes.

Times have changed. Now the profession is starting to pick up on Ezekiel's lenses. A leading authority on the oxygen transmissibility of materials recently tested the process and found that the gas permeable scleral lens provides five times more oxygen to the eye than it actually needs. Leading English eye hospital, Moorfields, has described Ezekiel's lens as the best lens for the cone-shaped eye disease keratoconus.

With the assistance of a $308,750 grant from the Industry Research and Development Board, Ezekiel and his optometrist son Damon are now developing a series of lenses to fit deformed or cone-shaped eyes. They are 'mapping' the eye, using instruments that give the shape of eyes, to evolve a series of fitting lens for various distorted eyes. This enables practitioners to give a patient a very close fit requiring minimal adjustment, whereas normally patients with very distorted eyes require a number of adjustments.

America, with a large and affluent population where one in 5000 suffers distorted or keratoconic eyes, is the obvious market place. The American Food and Drug Administration (FDA) fast-tracked approval of his lenses.

Ezekiel has also developed a gas permeable lens for babies who are born with cataracts, and this was a major factor in the fast tracking. Ezekiel says previous options for babies born with cataracts are not as effective, and the FDA said they "must have his lenses". FDA approval opens the US market.

Ezekiel said that if he hadn't received the R&D grant he would probably still have proceeded to develop his specialist lens, but it would have taken a lot longer and others could have beaten him to it.

While Ezekiel is concerned first and foremost about helping people to see – he conducts free clinics around the globe – he knows he is in a profitable industry.

His company is already sending fitting sets off to the United States and a teaching video is getting worldwide exposure.

"The potential is huge and we are getting our marketing strategy in place. The dollars will come," Ezekiel says.

While his company, Benra Pty Ltd, employs 30 people at his laboratories in Perth, Ezekiel's focus is still on patients and solutions to problems. He says none of what he has done has been rocket science. "It's basic common sense that's good for people and good for eyes."

At a recent US clinic he met a patient who had an unsuccessful corneal graft. "He couldn't see and they were going to do another graft. With one of my lenses he read the bottom line. It's cases like this that make it all worthwhile."

Last year after 20 years of pursuing 'pure logic', not rocket science, Don Ezekiel was recognised with the award of the Member of the Order of Australia for his work.

Contact:
Don Ezekiel
Benra Pty Ltd
3 Hutton St
Osborne Park WA 6017
Tel: (08) 9443 4944
Fax: (08) 9443 4147

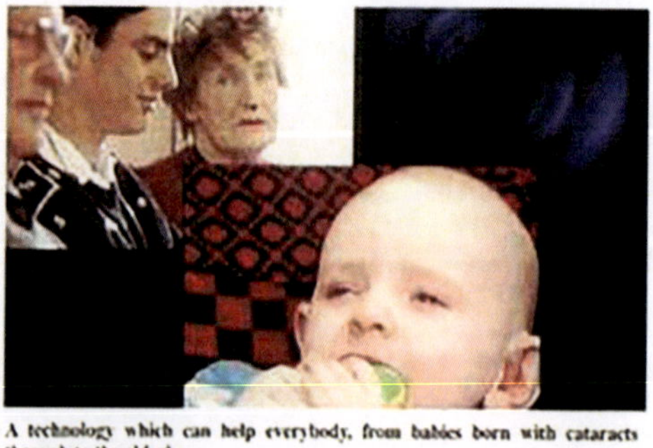

A technology which can help everybody, from babies born with cataracts through to the elderly.

ENTERPRISE

in his subject, when Ezekiel returned to Australia he felt that we were far behind the rest of the world. This led him to start his own contact-lens-making business and also to design and produce products such as hydrophilic extended wear contacts.

Although Ezekiel heads the company and leads research into new products, his Perth staff, led by group manager Barry Connell, turn the ideas into reality. "They are a superb staff," Ezekiel says.

The combination of Ezekiel's research and the manufacturing skills of his staff have led to the latest Gelflex breakthrough — a new type of intra-ocular lens that has drawn international attention. The product called Iogel, is an intra-ocular hydrogel lens implanted surgically in the eye.

Hailed as a forerunner of a new generation of lenses, Iogel is to be marketed worldwide through Alcon Laboratories on the US, part of the giant Swiss group, Nestle. World patents for the new lens have been applied for.

Ezekiel, as well as doing research at home, travels overseas regularly to keep abreast of world trends. On one of his recent trips he came close to disaster: he was at Rome airport minutes before the recent massacre. Sometimes he is accompanied on these trips by family members who offer advice on what they believe are fresh developments or matters worth enquiry. He regards the advice of his wife, Challis, as particularly important.

Ezekiel has never had professional business advice, although he has been well supported by his bank, the ANZ. Commenting on his overdraft, he says: "I think the bank really owns the business." However, he has not always enjoyed a good banking relationship.

The Perth end of the business specialises in the design and manufacture of contact lenses, most of which are exported. The Melbourne branch has expanded recently into bigger premises for the manufacture of sterile products for hospital and medical use. The new factory, at Dandenong, is believed to be the first to challenge foreign-owned manufacturers of the essential solutions.

Ezekiel discovered how strongly the multinationals were prepared to protect their market when he found himself in a price-cutting war for sterile intravenous solutions. But competition has not slowed plans for further expansion at the Dandenong factory, which is already employing about 25 people.

In the same way as he praises his Perth contact-lens workers, Ezekiel is equally impressed by his Melbourne staff. Commenting on one staff member who operates a plastic moulding unit, he says: "If he could take it to pieces and take it home he would sleep with it every night."

An indication of how thoroughly Ezekiel researches and plans his business is his establishment of a relationship with Alcon, the international marketer of his new lenses. Not until he was sure that his research and the work of Barry Connell had been completely successful did he select an overseas representative.

He says: "It then came time to contact Alcon, which I did late one night by telephone to the US. I was confident that we had a world-ranking product, but imagine trying to describe it over the phone.

"Anyway, it took the people at Alcon only a few minutes to realise that I was describing something special. They wanted me to fly immediately to the US to show them. 'No,' I said. 'I want you to choose your own technical specialist to come and see us and make an assessment.' Ten days later Alcon had one of the world's leading experts in Perth checking us out and now we have a deal by which lenses made in WA will be exported worldwide."

TIM TREADGOLD

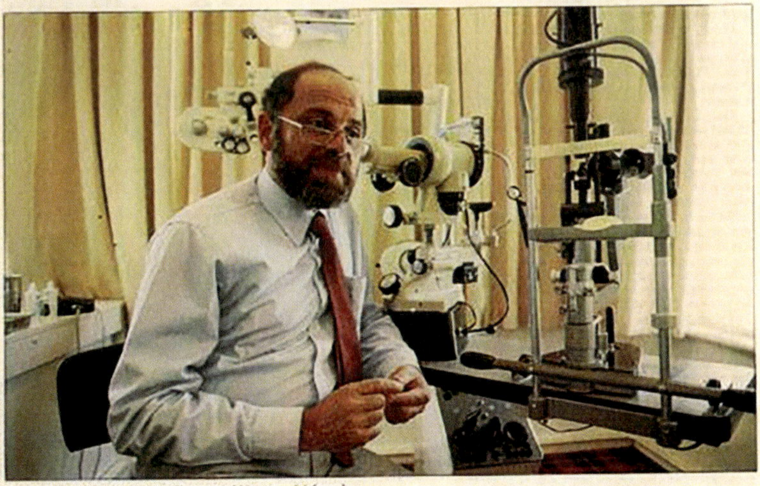

Donald Ezekiel: Having good staff is part of his successful formula

FEBRUARY 7, 1986, BUSINESS REVIEW WEEKLY 83

APPENDIX 7.

UNIVERSITY OF WA HONORARY DOCTORATE ACCEPTANCE SPEECH

Chancellor, Vice-Chancellor, Members of the Senate, distinguished guests, members of the staff, graduating class of 2023 and their guests, ladies and gentlemen.

I would like to express my deepest gratitude to the University of Western Australia. I can't begin to tell you how delighted I was to receive a letter a few months ago informing me of the University's decision to confer this honour upon me – an honorary doctorate is indeed most humbling and much appreciated.

My congratulations to the graduating class of 2023, with a special greeting to today's optometry graduates from someone who graduated from this wonderful university some 66 years ago. Back then I could never have imagined to be a recipient of an honorary doctorate, standing here and sharing such a memorable moment with you all today.

The visionaries who established this world-class faculty are to be congratulated. How fortunate you are to be the first graduates with an optometric doctoral degree from the University of Western Australia.

As graduates, your journey does not end today, it is truly just beginning. Although it may not seem so at the moment, what you have endured and accomplished is quite profound and of major significance to your future endeavours.

Woody Allen said, "It's clear the future holds great opportunities. It also holds pitfalls. The trick is to avoid the pitfalls, seize the opportunities - and get home by 6 o'clock."

I have had an interesting and fortunate life which became a life dedicated to the world of contact lenses.

This is a part of my journey.

I was born in Singapore to parents who were both refugees. My mother from Germany, my father from Iraq. When Singapore fell in 1942 our family became refugees and we managed to get on a hospital ship which brought us to our new home in Australia.

In 1953 I enrolled in the optometry course here at University of Western Australia.

Our pathology lecturer was ophthalmologist Ken Bardon-Brown. Ken trained in London and was fitting patients with glass scleral lenses. During his lectures he described the visual results obtained with this amazing lens for patients he had seen the previous week, just not possible with any other lens.

This was my introduction to contact lenses.

My father was an optometrist who stressed to me that the world was becoming a world of specialisation and I should look for a specialty. Contact lenses became my specialty.

I started fitting contact lenses after graduating and spent a month in Sydney with prominent optometrist Lloyd Hewett, who taught me his method of fitting scleral lenses.

I was fortunate to meet and marry a lovely girl who supported me in all my ideas, endeavours and achievements, which would not have otherwise been possible without her. Thank you Challis. I share this award with you.

Challis and I travelled to London for me to sit for postgraduate degrees and to gain experience, at a time when contact lenses were rapidly evolving.

The contact lens clinic at Moorfield's Eye Hospital exposed me to a large number of ocular conditions I had only read about in text books, and provided me with the opportunity to work and learn from some of the most remarkable specialists and researchers in the field of contact lenses – including Dame Ida Mann, who was the first female professor of ophthalmology and a senior surgeon at the Moorfield's Eye Hospital.

Ida moved to Perth in 1947. I was fortunate to know her well and some years later was privileged to unveil the blue plaque at her old London home where she was born.

Ida was awarded honorary doctorates by the University of Western Australia and Murdoch University, and was instrumental in establishing the Perth Lions Eye Institute. I am honoured to be walking in her footsteps today.

While in London, looking to gain experience, I went to the West End, came across an optical shop, Hamblins and applied for a position. I was told that their contact lens clinic was opposite and advised that the head of the clinic, a Josef Dallos, was a difficult man to work with and rarely employed people, preferring to work alone. At the interview I told him of my experience in fitting all types of lenses to which he replied "You don't know anything, I will teach you"... and offered me a job. I called my lecturer from the contact lens course at City University, Bob Fletcher, told him Dallos had offered me a position. I asked Bob if Dallos would he be a good person to learn from. He told me to "open your contact lens text book and read the first page".

There with a detailed description of his pioneering work was the "legend of contact lenses", Joseph Dallos.

Dallos was a warm person and a great teacher always telling me "whatever you do, you can always do better."

In 1971 I established a contact lens practice and returned to London every year to update on the evolving lens developments in contact lenses.

On a visit to Dallos he said to me "If you really care for your patients, you should make your own lenses and undertake research to test your ideas." He convinced me to do so and I ordered the equipment to make contact lenses. He also taught me how to research.

Eight months after the equipment arrived, when I was still learning how to make a decent lens, I received a high court writ from a New York company, advising me I was infringing on patents they owned. Papers from concerned stakeholders worldwide demonstrating that there was prior knowledge of their patent claims were received, proving they were not novel. My attorney replied to the patent office and nothing further was heard.

This was my introduction to patents and what companies do to protect their market.

It turned out to be a good learning experience.

Having a busy contact lens practice and a lens manufacturing facility, I became involved in research. Following a lecture I gave to ophthalmological registrars, one asked if I could make him an intraocular lens out of a soft contact lens material. I asked how many do you want? "If it works thousands, maybe millions".

That registrar was Graham Barrett, who is now an associate professor of ophthalmology.

Graham's design was complex and not possible to make with the equipment we had at the time so the design was modified and we made the world's first foldable intraocular lens out of a hydrogel material that needed just a small incision to implant the lens.

We applied for a patent which was granted in 1980. I must have learned.

Now what do we do?

The world's largest ophthalmic company was Alcon, a part of Nestle. They did not have an intraocular lens. I made one phone call and obtained the direct phone number of the president of Alcon, Tim Sear. I called Tim in Fort Worth and told him of the intraocular lens we had developed here in Perth.

With the help of a Harvard graduate friend living in America, an agreement with Alcon was made that included we manufacture the initial 5,000 lenses here in Perth, together with a very good royalty.

Unfortunately, the royalties never eventuated as Alcon subsequently acquired several intraocular lens laboratories, one of which had developed a new, better material for the intraocular lens, so understandably they moved to the new material.

When Tim visited us I asked what he had thought when he received my call regarding the intraocular lens. He replied that Alcon had a large office in Sydney and believed they knew everything that was happening in Australia, but when I said I was in Perth, Tim said, and I quote, " the buggers have probably done it".

To manufacture and package the lenses for use in the United States, the laboratory needed FDA approval. Alcon sent their Quality Assurance people to Perth and helped us to receive FDA approval to manufacture medical devices.

Some years later the Lions institute developed a material for an artificial cornea and asked us to shape the material to allow it to be transplanted to a human eye. This we did and developed a method by freezing the material to manufacture and provide artificial corneas for the Lions group to successfully implant to patients. It was a fascinating time where I learned more than I ever imagined a little contact lens practitioner and manufacturer in Perth was destined to.

Contact lenses have also exposed me to some of life's most wonderful situations.

When the World Series Cricket came to Australia, prominent Pakistani cricketer Madjid Khan made a century in every match played on the east coast. He lost a contact lens in Adelaide and consulted me when the team came to Perth. I prescribed and made him a new pair of contact lenses.

Can you see where this is going.?

In the Perth test ... Madjid made two ducks.

Thus ended my short career as the "possible" 13th man for Australian cricket.

Many projects I was involved in were not successful but every one of them provided something I learned from.

I kept progressing with my research and focused my efforts on two pioneering research areas:

gas permeable scleral lenses, and

a soft bifocal contact lens that provides clear vision at far and near without compromise, described as the holy grail of contact lenses.

Both have represented the greatest and most satisfying challenges of my career.

I am probably best known for my pioneering of the gas permeable scleral lens.

As you know, the scleral lens is often the only contact lens for patients with a range of pathological corneal problems to obtain vision. The lens is a comfortable lens for patients as it sits on the insensitive sclera and clears the sensitive cornea with the patient's tears neutralising all corneal distortions that affect their vision.

The scleral lens was not widely available to patients worldwide.

My pioneering of the gas permeable scleral lens came about through necessity.

Mary Bremner, senior ophthalmologist at Princess Margaret Children's Hospital, knew the benefits scleral lenses provided for patients. Mary would phone asking me to attend theatre and fit a scleral lens to a four-week old baby she had removed a cataract from. I would go the hospital, gown up and take an impression of the baby's eye, a method Dallos pioneered.

When the eye closes, Bells Phenomime occurs where the eye rolls up as a protective mechanism, resulting in my taking an impression of the lower canthus and little of the all-important cornea. This made fitting a lens hard on the baby, hard on their parents - and hard for me! There had to be a better way.

As there are no blood vessels in the cornea which would obstruct the passage of light to the receptors in the retina, its oxygen needs come directly from the air and from patients' tears.

Scleral lenses were made from glass or PMMA, materials which are impermeable to oxygen, BUT corneal lenses were now being fabricated from gas permeable materials. It was logical that gas permeable materials should be used for scleral lenses.

We were sourcing GP materials from Polymer Technology Corporation in Boston. I flew to Boston and met with the then owners Lou Major and Perry Rosenthal. Perry was senior ophthalmologist and head of contact lenses at the Massecuites Eye and Ear Hospital. He asked why I wanted large blanks, and I replied to use to make scleral lenses.

Perry retorted that no-one fitted scleral lenses anymore. I told him this was not correct, as a handful of practitioners worldwide offered this lens to patients, I being one, and from experience in practice and working with Dallos the scleral lens was the only lens able to help many ocular conditions.

A gas permeable lens would be healthier for the eye and maybe would be an easier lens for practitioners to fit, resulting in the lens being more readily available for patients.

They eventually agreed, sending me a rod of large diameter gas permeable material and I started fitting patients with gas permeable scleral lenses.

At the 1983 meeting of the British Contact Lens Association, I described the fitting of forty-three patients with a range of pathological conditions with scleral lenses manufactured from a gas permeable material. This was the first time a gas permeable scleral lens had been described.

The discussion at the meeting and later published in the contact lens press reported "the consensus was that no-one believed the results due to the thickness of the lens; that a gas permeable material would make no difference to the transmission of oxygen to the cornea".

The world authority on the oxygen permeability of materials, scientist Irving Fatt, was at the meeting and asked me for lenses so he could calculate the amount of oxygen passing through the lens to the eye. He calculated that "the eye receives five times more oxygen than the cornea needs".

The paper was published and Perry called and visited me. I arranged for patients with a range of ocular conditions to be fitted with the GP lens with comfortable, optimal vision, just not possible with any other lens, for Perry to see.

Perry returned to Boston and established the "Boston Sight Scleral Lens Foundation" introducing the gas permeable scleral lens, which is now widely available in America. Prominent practitioners worldwide introduced the lens in their countries, making the lens generally available.

Roger Buckley, Head of Moorfield's Eye Hospital, wrote to me in a personal letter, "the gas permeable lens is the medical contact lens par excellence. There is no eye shape that cannot be fitted with this type of lens".

Conferences are held and international contact lens journals are published, just on lens.

Dallos was right when he said, "anything and everything is possible".

A project to develop a soft bifocal lens that provides clear vision at both distance and reading, described as the "holy grail of contact lenses", was implemented.

There are two basic designs for a bifocal contact lens:

- *One is of a simultaneous vision design where both distance and reading lens powers are presented in the pupil area of the eye simultaneously, resulting in compromised vision. Variations of this design are the only soft bifocal lens now available.*

- *The other design is an alternating vision translating bifocal lens, similar to the optics of a bifocal spectacle lens with the distance power at the top and the reading power at the bottom of the lens.*

The translating bifocal lens provided optical clarity at both far and near, without compromise, but was only available in a rigid corneal lens form.

From my visits to the major laboratories, I learned that they had all had tried to manufacture a soft translating bifocal lens but had failed and given up, telling me it could not be done.

A translating bifocal lens in a lathed form was developed, but today's market is for a mass-produced disposable lens. All the major companies I visited expressed interest in the lens but only if it could be cast moulded, the process used for the mass manufacture of disposable lenses. A cast moulding laboratory was established here in Perth and demonstrated that the cast moulding of a translating bifocal lens could be done – after all, "anything and everything is possible" But getting a product to market is another story.

So the lessons I have learned which I pass onto you.

- *Anything and everything is possible:*

- *You must keep pushing the boundaries because there is nothing unachievable;*

- *Believe in it yourselves; and*
- *If you have an idea, and you believe it is better than what is currently available, ask your laboratory to make it for you. If they won't oblige, then move to another laboratory!*

But other factors come into play that do not relate to what you have developed, including;

- *Company personnel protecting their positions*
- *The "not the invented here" syndrome comes into play*
- *Presenting your ideas to the most senior company person provides a chance that your proposals might proceed further*
- *It's a tough world out there. It is not easy.*

And as Sarah Bon Brannock wrote, "The world needs dreamers and the world needs doers, but above all, the world needs dreamers who do."

You may not progress along simple straight lines, but with determination you will make a contribution to the world, no matter how small or big that contribution may be, it will be your very own legacy, the most indelible of your steps along your journey.

Congratulations again on your graduations. My very best wishes for your future.

My sincerest thanks again to the university for this wonderful award. It is truly humbling and very much appreciated.

Thank you for listening and allowing me to share this very special moment with you.

9 780645 309751

Printed at Repro India Ltd.